We'll Show Them

To Juanita
with all good wishes

Alan Councell

We'll Show Them

Alan Counsell

Memory Lane

First published in Great Britain by Pearl Press

ISBN 978-1-908515-16-2

Printed and bound by Good News Books Ltd, Ongar, Essex, England.

My entire life is shared by my wife, Kathleen, my soul mate. She is my constant companion and always there to give me encouragement and confidence. Her constant reinforcement of all that is positive in life spurs me on and undoubtedly my work could never have begun without Kathleen's inspiration. It was her idea to write this book and my gratitude towards her knows no bounds, not just for her encouragement to write but for the wonderful life we share together.

Acknowledgements

I would like to express my thanks and appreciation to John Heaton who gave me the encouragement and confidence to seek publication and to Julia Noble of my publishers, Memory Lane, for her consistent energy, constant patience and professionalism which gave impetus to the book which, without her contribution could never have been completed.

CONTENTS

PREFACE

I need time each day to be alone to pray to my Heavenly Father for through prayer I gain strength, knowledge and direction. I know my Saviour, Jesus Christ, and try to follow His teachings and example in my dealings with my fellow men whilst living my daily life.

I am a member of The Church of Jesus Christ of Latter-Day Saints and try to live the principles and concepts of this, my religion. I am the product of the shaping of obedience to the laws and statutes of God and find joy and fulfillment in discovering and achieving potential and in progressing to become that which my Deity would have me be.

I make mistakes. I am far from perfect but I learn and grow daily from recognising my weaknesses and trying to correct them. I fail many times and failure makes me human – hence my need to be alone each day to pray.

My life is wonderfully rich in blessings and achievements but I do not take anything for granted. I know the things which are given so freely to me can all be taken away in a flash, so I value all that goes to make up my amazing life. I have so much to be thankful for.

psi

CHAPTER ONE

I was born in Blackburn in Lancashire in 1937. Apparently my birth was difficult and complicated and I acquired brain damage soon after my birth. I was brought up in a small terraced house in a cobbled street with my sister and three brothers. Blackburn was a mill town and one of my earliest memories is waking up each morning to the sound of iron and wooden bottomed clogs on the bleached white pavements below the bedroom window as the mill workers walked past our home on their way to work.

Because of the effects of cerebral palsy (brain damage), I was unable to walk until around nine years of age and unable to speak in a way others could understand until my teenage years. My childhood was a mixture of kindness from my extended family, ridicule from others and dramas ranging from my own temper tantrums, caused by severe frustration – the only means of gaining attention – to struggles against authorities who wanted to classify me as 'mental' or amputate my limbs because they thought artificial limbs would be more use to me than my own. I have nightmarish memories of being ridiculed, both in the street and at school by children who found me a great source of entertainment. What was maybe more embarrassing than the ridicule itself was the public nature of these daily incidents, or the memories of being called to the head mistress's office, never knowing why until I arrived at her desk – would it be another letter for my parents, which would send my dad into orbit? – a letter complaining about the state of my clothes because I dribbled so profusely, a letter recommending my right arm be amputated, or inviting me to attend a school for mental defectives.

Although my walking, my posture, the use of my hands and my speech were all affected by my brain damage, there was never anything wrong with my intellect. This was proven when I was expelled from mainstream school and offered a place at a school for mental defectives. My parents and grandparents,

1

along with help from our family doctor, fought this and this episode in my life culminated in my attendance at a mental health tribunal where I was pronounced to be of sane mind and an above average intelligence. I was very aware of all the negative messages given to me during my formative years. I wasn't acceptable the way I was – I had to change and become like others!

Through willpower and sheer bloody-mindedness I forced myself to walk, ignoring the advice of the medical profession. Reading and writing were difficult and speech was a mammoth undertaking but with the help of my family, friends and neighbours I achieved the impossible. Impossible – because before I reached my second birthday my parents were told I would never walk or talk and there was a possibility I would be uneducable. They were also told I would not live beyond the age of ten.

The effects of all the negatives of my childhood were devastating. I internalised all of the oppressive, degrading and inhuman treatments and comments of my young life and in my late teens found relief and blissful oblivion in alcohol. I became an alcoholic. In drink I found I was released from thoughts of inadequacy, from debilitating shyness and a severe lack of confidence, from shaky dexterity, and became unaware of my communication problems. It was my friend Eileen who recognised my drink problem and worked so hard to get me off the bottle. Eileen and I went to school together and we became inseparable, maybe because she experienced similar problems, because she had a glandular problem and appeared very grossly overweight. We both worked at the same cotton mill when we left school and it was when she discovered my flask of coffee actually contained alcohol that she became alerted to my problem. She also followed me to the pub at lunchtime and again in the evening. Eileen and I had physical fights over my addiction. She also enlisted the help of two other friends. Between them they made me see the error of my ways and it took a great strength of will on my part to give up alcohol. I soon realised that alcohol only masked the problem temporarily. The problems were still there when I was sober; alcohol didn't cure anything. In the cold light of day I had to live and accept myself for who I was and what I was. I had to decide whether to live my life as best I could or drown myself in the expensive oblivion of alcohol.

I think my problems were impacted because I could not actually speak during my early life and so could never verbalise my feelings. I was cared for remarkably well by each member of my immediate family and many of my extended family but I think there is a verbal reasoning power that develops along with the comprehension and expression of language and I didn't possess this verbal reasoning as a child. Not being able to express my thoughts, feelings and not being able to reply and respond verbally to what was happening in my life compounded the damage.

It has been a continuing fight throughout my life for acceptance and to be treated as ordinary. That fight still goes on today! I had to work really hard to overcome the difficulties imposed by acquiring the crucial skills of mobility and speech (and thus thought) at a late stage in life. Many people worked with me in my acquiring of these skills and although I am intensely shy and face prejudice I feel indebted to those wonderful people and feel I must achieve all I can in life and live it to the full.

As I reflect on life, I am awestruck by my successes and achievements. I have worked well beyond the expected years, well beyond retirement age. I am married to an adorable, admirable and beautiful wife. I have reared three absolutely sensational children (I even have grandchildren). I have attended college and university and have a stream of academic qualifications. I have held senior positions in the health and education sector and since 1990 have run a successful training and consultancy business. Maybe those who criticised, ridiculed, oppressed and rejected me in early life did more good than harm. Maybe they taught me and gave me a personal strength that has made me extraordinarily determined and has aided development and achievement.

Mother

It would seem that mum was singled out to be my mum. No other woman could have coped so intelligently with all the problems I had in life and no other could have supported, cared and encouraged as she did.

What a shock it must have been to give birth and have a disabled child. I was the fifth child born to my parents and traditionally mum had had relatively easy births. From the little I know of my birth it was excruciating and long for my mum. I was born in the breech position and usually this is anticipated before the birth but apparently in my case it was totally unexpected. I cannot imagine what mum must have endured to give me life. Even after the birth it must have been traumatic because I had great difficulty in breathing and was resuscitated by our family doctor more than once in the first twenty four hours of life. That's how my brain was damaged! During my first hours of life my brain was deprived of oxygen as I stopped breathing and some of the brain

3

cells were damaged.

I am told that feeding was a real problem because my sucking reflex was so weak. For the first four months of my life I was fed with an eye dropper. It must have been a full time job – maybe it took all day to feed me. Most of the family were involved along with my grandparents and several neighbours as well. I became more reliable at the age of four months and was able to feed from a bottle.

Mother was forty years of age when I was born, and was a really good looking woman. She had very long chestnut brown hair that shone like the feathers of a raven. So long was her hair, she was able to sit on it. She would plait her hair each day and coil it in a bun at the nape of her neck whilst she worked in the family bakehouse and while doing her domestic chores. At other times she would wear her hair in a pigtail or a ponytail hanging down her back. I think mother's eyes were her best feature; they were a grey-blue and conveyed warmth and communicated a wealth of varying emotions. Looking at her eyes, one could readily tell if she was angry or disappointed with you. Her eyes would convey compassion, concern, support and genuine love that eased the hurt and devastating moments of my young life. One look could wither but another could give confidence and support or take away the hurt from a hostile world. Mother also had a mischievous streak and a sense of humour that made her eyes twinkle and dance.

Mum did not marry until the age of twenty-five and it is said that mum and dad knew each other while they were in school. Mum left school at the age of twelve and went to work as a weaver in a cotton mill. Both mum and dad lived the whole of their lives in the Audley district of Blackburn. Mum attended the Ranters church in the early years of her life but apparently the local church closed down during the First World War and mum did not attend church after that time

As a family I think we benefited from mother's religious philosophy. It was an unwritten family law that each of us had to be in the house for Sunday tea. Even my dad had to be home from his working men's club, his only social outing in the week. Woe betide anyone who was missing! At four-thirty every Sunday the front door was locked; at other times the front door was always unlocked and neighbours and others would open the door, shout 'hello' or 'are you there?' and walk in. Sometimes it was like living in Piccadilly Circus, a constant stream of visitors, none invited but all welcomed.

But Sunday afternoon we were all together as a family and the rest of the world was locked out. There were always homemade fancy cakes and home-baked fruit pies for tea and these would be spread, nay, displayed on silver coloured and glass cake stands and decorated china plates on mum's best white cloth with the elaborate crochet edging on the dining table. The same things happened each week: dad would tell us a 'proverb'. He wouldn't read it from the Bible; he would tell it in his own words and the family would discuss it. Then mum would tell of neighbours who needed help, assign one or two of us to give that help and then she always commented on how each member of the family had helped another member of the family. I can remember the good feeling in our home each Sunday as we all came together – lots of fun and laughter, besides the serious stuff, and lots of family hugs too. Mum was very keen on us helping each other and helping others outside the family as well. Her words were, 'If you see a need in others try to help, if you see someone struggling or having a problem, be there for them. We are a family and we should always be there for each other.' Mum would often ask us, 'What good turn have you done today?' She would ask my dad as well! She used to say, 'If you think about others and their needs, you won't be selfish or ungrateful, nor dwell too much on your own problems. Giving is better than taking because it makes you happy and makes you aware of what you have to give and how rich we are, not in money but in ability, in health and compassion. You always learn something from helping others – something about yourself and about others. Usually selfishness leads to unhappiness. If you can think of others and help them, your own problems will seem small and you will feel good about yourself!' My mother was a remarkable woman. She worked with my dad in the family bakehouse, which was located next door to our home, from 4 a.m. each morning. None of us, her family, went to school or work without a cooked breakfast and we also had a cooked lunch and more often than not a cooked meal in the evening. She baked all her own bread too.

Mum ruled her family with a rod of iron. There were so many of us and she was a busy person and we had to have discipline in the family. But she was always fair and just and because every one knew the limits and boundaries we were a very happy family.

Alker Street was a community all on its own: the neighbours shared each other's lives, they shared each other's joys and happiness, problems and grief and they felt each other's pain. We were intrinsically connected to each other.

I would suggest that within each of us there is a need to feel that we belong. Our neighbours, throughout my young life were always there for me, they always had time for me. I remember being surrounded by happy people. The neighbours were like an extended family, always there for each other, unselfish and willing never looking for praise or recognition but always helping each other and through their example and mother's encouragement I was taught to have concern for my fellow men!

Father

Father was a giant of a man. He was very powerfully strong and muscular. He was about six feet three inches in height and almost as broad as he was long. His neck measurement was twenty inches. He was so strong! He volunteered for the army at sixteen, lying about his age, and served with the Enniskillen Fusiliers in the 1914-18 war. He was gassed by mustard gas whilst serving in the trenches and this affected his lungs and his heart for the rest of his life.

I'm a little confused about dad's religion. All his family attended the Church of England but it is said that dad attended The Ranters Church before he joined the army! However, on his return from the army in 1920 dad did not want anything to do with religion of any kind and although he would never tell anyone of his time in the army, he did say, 'I've seen awful things happen to the nicest of men. I cannot understand how there can be a God. If there was a God, how could he allow to happen what I saw?!' If he were challenged in any way by anyone he would become angry and say, 'Go away and witness and experience what I have, then come back and talk to me about God.'

Certainly, I witnessed the noise from his nightmares, which occurred frequently through out his entire life, as he relived his experiences in the trenches as he served his country.

He never stopped his family from attending church and one could talk to him about churchy things but he would never give an opinion on any doctrine. He always said his religion was the way he lived and the way he treated other people.

Dad always said he had become a 'humanist' rather than a member of any religion and he used philosophy rather than religious doctrine to govern his behaviour. He had a particular system and a very personal set of beliefs based on his experience of human behaviour. He would talk about the camaraderie and the trust he found amongst the men he served with in the army. He told us that if he could get that camaraderie and that trust in his family he would have succeeded in life.

I think dad must have had a good knowledge of the Bible, for he often quoted it in teaching us how to behave. He seemed to be particularly fond of the Book of Proverbs. I often wonder if he knew it by rote. He used to say the answers to many of life's problems lay in the wisdom of King Solomon!

As a family we were certainly exposed to many of the Proverbs. Father seemed to recite a proverb and ask, 'What does that mean to you?' I still remember being taught about pride, morality, friendship and how to speak to people. Father seemed to have a knack of using Proverbs to teach his family how to live. We, as a family, were taught about pride and being grateful. We were taught about being cheerful, happy and having a sense of humour. Father's philosophy wasn't shared with us from any religious orientation but from a behavioural point of view. Father had a slant on life which stemmed from his concern for his family and his fellow men rather than divine or religious matters.

Although I consider myself to be religious, most of dad's teachings from my childhood have stayed with me and have added to my life. Many times my behaviour has been modified as I have remembered the teachings of my dad from my younger years.

Basically dad was a very kind man and very family orientated. He was always there for his family. He worked as a crumpet maker in the family business. The bakehouse was next door to our family home and dad worked all hours of the day and night. Many times in a week he would start baking crumpets maybe at nine in the evening and work through the night. Then he would deliver to his regular customers and hawk the remainder of his crumpets from door to door during the day. So dad got all kinds of visitors in the bakehouse. If a neighbour had an emergency during the night they would go to the bakehouse, dad would wake mum and together they would help with the emergency.

It could have been said that dad had a bad temper and used a lot of swear words but his family were very aware of how hard he worked and what little sleep he got. His sleep was often interrupted by his nightmares too. So we understood him. Mostly his tempter was directed at people who 'put me down'.

It was seldom that dad took a day from work but occasionally he would take us to Blackpool for the day. I would be carried on his shoulders and would put my arms around his forehead because my balance was non-existent – I had to 'hang on tight'. As I got older and more aware of myself, maybe around eight years of age, I noticed that whilst I was being carried on his shoulders I was dribbling on his head. This disturbed me and somehow I managed to communicate my concern to dad. I'll never forget his response. 'Alan, you're my son! I love carrying you around! Don't you ever be ashamed of something you can't help! I don't mind your dribble, it wipes off with a towel!' I remember that towel. It was used to cocoon me on the beach. I would be totally enveloped in this soft, snowy white towel to protect my clothes whilst dad fed me the biggest ice cream he could buy.

Throughout the many traumas of my young life dad was always there for me – always my champion and protector! He instilled in me the notion of individuality as he used to frequently say, 'Your life is not going to be like others but you do have a life. Live it!' After each of the many confrontations with various authorities he would always lift me from my feet, give me a rib-crushing hug and say, 'Silly buggers! We'll show them. You'll prove the buggers all wrong. I know you will.' (No one could give a hug like my dad! He comforted, protected, strengthened and conveyed loving acceptance through his hugs!)

Those three words, 'We'll show them!' have remained with me throughout my life and have often been repeated in my mind. They have spurred me on during low and difficult times and have heightened the excitement and feelings of achievements. They are a constant reminder that I have exceeded the low expectations of my young life and that I have actually proved the 'buggers' wrong.

My Siblings

Maybe many of us know something of the courage it takes for one to stand in opposition to tradition, custom or belief. None of us likes to be ridiculed. Daily, during my childhood, I experienced public ridicule and bullying from other children and degradation, humiliation and oppression from adults, professionals and the establishment. It seemed to be the custom if not the tradition in my young days to target 'the cripple' as my peers named me. It seemed I had to conform to acceptable norms or I was damned and wicked. Everyone commented on what I couldn't do and tried to change me or punish me.

My sister and brothers gave me the courage to go on. It was as though someone had explained my problems to them and they were the therapy I needed. They too faced ridicule because of their 'crippled brother' but each was loyal to me. I think there are few who are able to withstand popular opinion even as adults, even when they know that opinion is wrong, but my sister and brothers had physical fights with others in defending me. It would have been far easier for them to have joined the mob in bashing the cripple than defending him. It is difficult for me to comprehend the magnificent courage required by my sister and brothers in physically supporting me throughout my young life. Each of my siblings had a life and friends of their own but also found the time for me.

My next older brother, Joe, was three and a half years older than me and when I was five he would carry me to school each day on his back. He was not even nine years of age and he carried me to school in the morning, home again for lunch, back to school after lunch and home again at the end of the school day. The journey from home to school was about three quarters of a mile! If I needed the toilet whilst at school Joe would be sent for and he would carry me to the toilet. Sometimes I would have 'an accident' whilst in school, because not having speech made it difficult to express my needs and Joe would be sent for to carry me home. So he witnessed and also became a victim of the incessant daily ridicule and bullying I received, because I was always being carried by him. Never once did I ever hear him complain or murmur. Occasionally he would retaliate and get into fights and receive bloodied noses and other injuries but never did he say he was not going to carry me. On reflection, I don't know how he did it. He had a heavy load in more ways than one. Joe and I were inseparable until he was conscripted into the Army aged 18.

I experienced an agonising and debilitating loneliness when Joe left home for his conscripted two years in the Army. I was not aware of how I depended on him. I became a lost soul without him. Ultimately though, I'm sure it was good for my overall development to live for two years without the support of my big brother!

We were lifelong friends and during the last two years of his life on earth we texted or spoke together everyday. Boy! How I miss him.

My sister, Olive, was twelve years of age when I was born and when I was three and a half my younger brother, Tom, was born. At this time Olive was working full time but she used to come home from work and take over my care as mother's priorities were the new baby's needs. Olive was a fun person and even to this day, whenever we are together, we giggle. I was fed by Olive whenever she was home and feeding me was not an easy task but somehow this young teenager, my sister, had the skill and the knowhow to help me to swallow, which was really difficult for me to do. Later in my childhood she taught me how to chew, another function I had great difficulty with. In retrospect, I am awestruck at the patience displayed by Olive; she was like a

9

second mother to me. She gave me so much time and put so much effort into looking after me and it was all made so much fun. We laughed and giggled all the way through my early problems. Later on in her teenage years Olive went out in the evening with friends, and they would go dancing or to the cinema. But always would I be fed, bathed and put to bed by her before she went out. Even though mum had time to do these things as my baby brother got older, Olive would always insist. Olive and I have always been friends and have shared so much together. Today, even though we live miles apart, we speak to each other on the telephone at least three times a week. How fortunate I am to have a sister named Olive.

John, my eldest brother, was nine when I was born and I look upon him as my inventive brother. I remember him inventing games for me to play when I was quite young. I don't want to spoil his macho image but he was so sensitive and caring. He was a choir boy in a church choir and from an early age he would comfort me by taking me into his arms and singing to me, very softly. When I began school he was 13 years of age and had just started work. Joe would tell him all about my day – the ridicule and bullying – and John would always find a quiet corner and play with me on his return from work. He would always tell me how great I was and how well I was doing and he would often cry and tell me he had to go to work but wished he could come to school with me to protect me and sort 'them' out.

Throughout my younger years John was always there to encourage and support me. I think John was the one who got me walking. For a brief few months before he was conscripted into the Army at eighteen years of age, he spent time physically supporting me whilst my legs were strong enough to allow me to walk. He would massage my legs and sing as we practiced walking. Joe and Olive were also involved in teaching me to walk, as were my parents and some of my aunts, but I remember how John responded to my 'outbursts' and my insistence as I became obsessed with walking. He was so kind and gentle.

John always kept in touch with me throughout his short life. He died at the age of 48. He rejoiced at my every achievement and although he was a big, strong macho male, he was the one who cried the most at my wedding.

John chose to serve with the Royal Corps of Signals when called into the Army and spent most of his time in Palestine!

During his time in the Middle East there was much trouble and I think British Troops were there as a peacekeeping force. John was a despatch rider! He was always fond of motor bikes.

10

One day he and a colleague were sent on despatches together. Although they were in a war zone, the immediate area had been clear of action for a few weeks. Being young men and riding on an open road through the desert, they decided to race from A to B. John's companion is said to have got about ten feet in front of John. Suddenly John saw the other rider fall from his bike and he also saw something fly through the air! John was able to avoid the other rider and his bike which had fallen in his path by slowing down very quickly and swerving off the road. John approached his mate, the other rider, very cautiously. He found a headless body! The thing John had seen flying through the air had been his mate's head! A wire had been stretched between two poles hidden in the sparse vegetation across the road, meant to dismount despatch riders. So taut was the wire, it had decapitated John's companion. Obviously the wire was at the right height to catch this young man in the region of his throat! Had John been in the lead, who knows the consequences!?

John returned home after his demob and he was an absolute wreck. He greeted each member of the family with a long, drawn-out hug and he seemed to keep it together! When my turn came for a hug, he broke down and wept, and through his tears he mumbled, 'I thought I'd never see you again!' and he hugged me very tightly and he wept!

Dad separated us, took John into his arms and tried to comfort him.

After a long period of time dad released John from his hold, turned to mum and said, 'Can we cope if I take a few days off work?'

'We'll manage somehow!'

'Right then, I'd like to take John away for a few hours. Can you have two beds made up in the front parlour for when we get back?'

'They may have to be makeshift. They may have to be made up on the floor. Will that do?'

'Aye. That'll do. I'm not going to leave his side for a few days!'

Dad and John left the house and returned much later. Apparently John was very drunk! Dad apologised to mum and said he thought John needed a good, long sleep and that he thought drink might induce that much-needed sleep.

Dad took a few days from work, which had never been known before, and he stayed by John's side. Even when dad returned to work he took John with him! They were together for around seven weeks. During that time John had one nightmare where he relived the horrors of his time in the forces. Somehow dad had talked him through these horrors and helped John recover. No one in the family ever knew how dad had helped John but ironically dad

11

continued to relive the horrors of his time in the trenches through periodic nightmares!

John was able to return to work as a welder after being released from the Army after ten weeks.

I remember one occasion in my life when I was a young man. I received a severe telling off from John. He had taken his wife and family to the Blackpool illuminations and invited me along too. As we drove back in his car, he stopped at a fish and chip restaurant for supper. At the time I was very self conscious and avoided the 'public' as much as possible. It could also have been that I had never eaten in a public restaurant without my parents before. Eating was also difficult. I had to concentrate on so many things whilst eating. Shaky hands made it difficult to get the food into my mouth, limited arm movement didn't help and chewing and swallowing did not come naturally – I really had to concentrate. I was also prone to 'choking' and sometimes coughed and spluttered when I tried to swallow. So I wasn't comfortable eating in public. I hesitated over my fish and chips and John became angry with me and said, 'Alan, you're not eating because you think others are looking at you! Am I right?' I nodded. John continued, 'Well, do you know something? You're good enough to be looked at! The people who look at you might be admiring you! Be proud of yourself. I could never have done what you have. You've worked so hard. Now eat, enjoy, you deserve your fish and chips more than anyone else in this restaurant.' The memory of those remarks and this kind of encouragement, have strengthened me throughout my life.

My younger brother Tom did all he could but, being the youngest, he was kind of swamped by my older siblings. Nonetheless, he was always there for me. I do have a secret regret where Tom is concerned. I regret not being able to be the big brother he should have had and I do have a little feeling of guilt as I may have taken some attention away from him as a youngster as the rest of the family cared for me. Tom and I have always been and still are good friends!

I do not know how my family coped with all the trauma of my early years. They were supportive of each other and supportive of me. My father was leader of the pack and he led by example. My mother was supportive of my father and we all followed father's advice and counsel. We were united and had a great sense of family. There are principles from the success of my father's leadership which I have adopted in my own family, as a husband and a father, which have also helped me through my work years, particularly now as I run my own business. The successful leader, be it in the family or in business, has got to have a sincerity of purpose and has to carry through that which he says;

Saying one thing and, doing another does not work!

It would have been so easy for my family to ostracise me. I had very limited ability in every area of life but I was always included in every family activity and many domestic tasks too. As a family, we often played board games like Snakes and Ladders, Ludo and Draughts. I could not handle or manage the small container for shaking the dice, which came with the game, so we used a large mug, in Lancashire called a pint pot, to 'throw' the dice. Both of my hands were placed around the mug and I would shake the dice and tip them out of the mug. In Ludo, I would choose which counter I wanted moved and someone would move it for me, the same when we played draughts. Someone would move my draughts as I indicated. Eventually, John taught me to hold a pencil between my teeth and I was supported as I leaned over the draught board and indicated with my pencil where I wanted my move to be.

I remember playing cards with my family too. John produced a large scrubbing brush so I could place my hand of cards in its bristles. I would choose the card I wanted to play using my teeth and each time I would be reminded to swallow before I chose a card, then I wouldn't dribble and wet the cards.

These 'family games' took much longer to complete with me involved than ordinarily and I do wonder where the family got their patience from.

Similarly, family members were assigned chores each week, particularly on a Saturday morning, and I remember being involved. We had a 'fire range' in the living room (a coal fire with oven attached). Each Saturday morning in winter time the fire would burn very low and in summer time the fire would be extinguished. The oven interior was swept and washed. The outside of the oven door, the fire grate and surround had to be painted with 'black lead' and the brass bits polished. Often I would be involved in this. I was supported because I couldn't stand and the person supporting me would hold my wrist and guide my hand as I painted the oven door or applied 'Brasso' to the brass hinges and handle on the door. It would have been easier for the assigned person to do it themselves but I was always involved, it was always fun and I was always praised for my effort. Another chore I was always involved in was 'wet stoning' the front door step and widow bottom. This meant the doorstep was thoroughly washed and, whilst it was still wet, rubbed with a piece of 'sandstone'. This gave the step colour. I was able to do this almost on my own. I had to be supervised because my balance, even on all fours, wasn't great and I could easily fall over.

In the bakehouse, the hotplate had to be cleaned. These hotplates were around 5' by 7' (1,5m x 2,1m) and the crumpets were baked on them. Each

Saturday morning they were sprinkled with gritty sand and a large flat stone was rubbed over them; the friction of the stone on the gritty sand removed grease from the hotplates and cleaned the surface. They were then swept, washed and dried and I was held in someone's arms and involved as much as possible in this cleaning process.

I suppose I could say I came from quite a musical family inasmuch as dad and my two older brothers had good singing voices and would often sing solos or duets or even all together to entertain the rest of the family. My brothers also played the spoons and 'rick-racks'. (Spoons were two tablespoons held with a finger between the handles, with the bowls back-to-back and tapped on the knee and thigh in such a way as to make a rhythmic clicking sound; rick-racks were two pieces of flat bone held in the hand with a finger between them and shaken in such a way as to create a clicking rhythm.) They also played mouth organs, bazookas, and combs and paper. Always did we have music in our home and even though we didn't have television we entertained each other. We also had a wind-up gramophone. John and Olive would move the furniture back and do the jitterbug, which was the dance craze of the 1940s.

We had a battery radio too and every evening the family would gather at 6:45 to listen to Dick Barton, Special Agent.

CHAPTER TWO

My secondary school was like my junior school except that it had two storeys. It had the same type of corridor which stretched its full length. From one side you could look out over a quadrangle and see the junior school. On the other side of the corridor were windows, from floor to ceiling, which allowed you to see into each classroom. People seemed to be interested in watching me write as I sat at a desk by the corridor window. 'What an oddity I must be' – they had never seen anyone using two hands to write before. I had been used to having the same teacher for all classes in my junior school, but now we had a different teacher every hour. No one had spoken to me yet and I felt terribly nervous, as I didn't know many of the children. Each teacher who came into the room stood and watched me work. I didn't know if they had been made aware of my problems. By now I had begun to be dimly aware of how destructively self-conscious I was. I used to laugh at all the wrong moments.

At breaktime I had to find my way into the playground and I was amazed at the number of other children walking along the corridor. As all of us had to go down the same staircase to get outside and to the toilets, I was frightened to go down with them in case I fell into the crowd. I felt rather shaky and alone because of all the newness and strangeness. I waited until most of the children had descended and then went down carefully holding on to the wall. This made some of the children laugh. Through the corridor windows they had already seen me writing and they began to ask me questions. They wanted to know why I came down the stairs so slowly and why I wrote the way I did. I was trying to explain to them but they thought my talking was hilarious. As I entered the playground, more children asked about my writing and they too find the way I speak funny. It is as much as I can do to stop myself crying. Finally playtime ended and everyone had to go back into school. Again I had not the confidence to climb the stairs with the crowd so I decided to visit the toilet and hoped that the stairs would be quieter when I had finished.

In the toilets I met a boy who had seen me in my classroom and he asked me why I wrote like that. I tried to explain but received a smack round the head and I was told that in future I would speak properly when I spoke to him. I felt like running home to my mother, but a teacher appeared to hurry us up. As I was climbing the stairs, feeling very hurt and sorry for myself, I was told to make haste by the teacher. Of course I was late for class and had to explain why.

This was difficult as I was also fighting back tears while I tried to talk. Obviously the teacher couldn't tell what I said and simply patted my head. I felt embarrassed and lost. I wished people could hear the words I spoke as I heard them; they were so clear to me.

On my way home from school for lunch I met Norman, an old friend from junior school. He was also attending the secondary school for the first time today and he chatted to me all the way home. I tried to explain how I felt. Although he could not understand much of what I was saying he got the word 'stairs' and by a process of my nodding and shaking my head to various questions he understood one of my problems. He arranged to be at the staircase whenever possible to help me up and down.

Norman became friendly with me during our last year in junior school when he was having difficulty in memorising his tables. I knew mine very well and as the other children were rather cruel to Norman, he asked if I would help him. As I spent my playtimes watching the others rather than joining in their games, I welcomed the activity of hearing Norman's tables. I used to try and correct him as he recited to me; although he had difficulty in understanding me, I may have helped him to learn, as I stopped him each time he went wrong. He became friendly to me in school and taught me to kick a ball. I used to fall on my backside each time I lifted a leg but Norman was patient. He was the first friend I ever had in school and I used to think about him all the time; he was very special to me. He had lots of other friends and they used to tease him about being friendly with me. I did not like it when he played games with them rather than being with me. I would have liked to join in their games but they were too rough and my brother wasn't around to help me. Maybe when some of the children in my new school saw how clever I was, they would be friends with me like Norman was.

I didn't really feel like going to school after lunch but mother would never allow me to stay home and Norman had called for me so that we could walk to school together. As we got to school we were met by a group of children who saw me at breaktime that morning and they were asking questions and were laughing at my efforts to answer. Mercifully the bell sounded for afternoon school. I had decided not to sit near the window as I did that morning. I sat on the opposite side of the room but there was a rumpus as the boy who this morning sat in the seat I had chosen wanted the same seat again and I had to return to my original desk. I tried to stay in the classroom during afternoon break but this was not allowed, so I locked myself in a toilet until it was time to return to class.

There was a group of children waiting for me at the close of school and they too found the way I spoke rather amusing. The journey home had never seemed so long. I was frightened of falling as I was jostled by the crowd. I was so glad to see mother and home seemed like a sanctuary. I tried to explain to mother what had happened during the day and how miserable I felt but she did not understand half of what I was saying and dismissed my tears by saying that I would eventually make friends.

I could not go to sleep when I went to bed and I lay scheming as to what I would do tomorrow. I was going to set out as if I were going to school, but make a detour so as to miss all the other children and spend the day in the park. If I didn't come home for lunch at the correct time, mother would know what I had done, but I knew where there was a clock. My plan worked very well. I had arrived home for lunch at the right time and felt relieved that I had not been found out. Mother asked me how school had been that morning. As I nod in reply a letter was thrust at me and as I read it I sensed mother's anger. The letter was from the headmaster telling mother of my absence from school, making sure that she knew I wasn't there. Someone delivered the letter before lunch. Of course the headmaster knew my parents well through my older brothers and sister, who all went to his school.

The headmaster waited for mother and me as we arrived at school after lunch. He took us to his study, where he asked me where I had been all morning and why.

The study is quiet and the head looked stern and he would not allow mother to answer for me. I had to tell him everything and he took great pains to understand what I was trying to say. Although I had to repeat my words many times, I couldn't remember anyone listening to me and wanting to understand me like this man did. He did not seem to care how many times I repeated things to him, he made me feel that he was interested and had time for me. He summarised what I had said to make sure that he had understood it correctly and then told me that the teaching staff were all aware of my problems and all they expect is that I did the best I could. The head's concern now was

17

that I had got behind in the tests we were having that week, which are to find out what stream we should go in. He thought I would need more time for them than the other children because yesterday I did not complete very much of the papers we were given. He invited me to work at a desk in his room until I had completed all of the tests, so that I would be placed in the correct stream. He also told me to go to him with any problems I might have in the future. As the afternoon was now almost finished, I was allowed to go home with my mother.

I thought I was lucky to have a headmaster who recognised that while I might have written slowly and with great difficulty, that did not necessarily mean that the papers and tests themselves were too hard for me.

As I worked in the head's room during the next three weeks finishing the tests, I was introduced to all the teachers and developed a relationship with the headmaster. There were times at break and when I was walking home that I was harangued by groups of children, but they did me no physical harm and I could bear their harassment because the head discussed it with me. He did not want to make a public announcement about my being in the school; he thought that might attract even more attention to me and that if I could ignore the comments and refuse to be hurt by them, the bullies would lose interest.

Now that I had completed all the tests I could be placed with a class. It was much better now that I was always with the same group of children and knew the teachers who took us for each subject. I was tolerated by the other children in my form and as they got to know me better they understood more of what I said.

At the end of the autumn term the school had a competition that each form had to enter. Each class had to produce a play and perform it in front of the whole school. I was certainly not equipped to participate in dramatics and I was wondering what I would be asked to do. I was hoping that I would be left out, but the headmaster had other ideas and insisted that I be stage manager for my form. For the first time I had been given responsibility and the staff really involved me.

In my second year I had an art teacher who had an unusual voice. I couldn't say he had a speech impediment but his voice was nasal and thick and he also had one arm that he could not straighten. He had difficulty using the hand of that arm. I had never been a success at art and hid away all my work. If I could, I threw it in the wastebin before anyone could see it. But this teacher encourages me and showed a book to the class. It contained pictures by a famous artist and the teacher was asking whose paintings they looked like. The other children seem to see a similarity between my work and the pictures in the book. The painting I had today was of a clown and I allowed the teacher to pin it up on the wall. It was the very first time any of my work had been displayed. Very slowly people seemed to be accepting me as I was and recognised that although I did not have their abilities, I might have others of my own. Knitting was one: I learned it from Mammy Brogden (a neighbour), and though others called it cissy, I enjoyed it. Father always wore my scarf, holes and all.

Try as I may I still could not swim. I had lessons at school and Harry, my sister Olive's husband, still took me swimming each Saturday morning but I could not control the rolling of my hips in the water. I had been unable to make any progress.

As the drama competition came round for the second time, I was sent for by the headmaster who suggested that I could write a play for my class to perform. I didn't really feel that I could do this but the headmaster was persuasive, so I had a try.

I wrote a play and called it The Rose-coloured Spectacles. It is a sort of fairy tale about a bad-tempered princess who is disliked by all her subjects and family; she is given a pair of rose-coloured spectacles which make her good-tempered and likeable, she meets her Prince Charming, marries him and lives happily ever after. The headmaster edited it for me and I noticed the number of corrections he made to the script. I was amazed that he never commented on any mistake but instead gave a lot of praise for the idea behind the script. My form produced it on stage and it was well received by the audience. But I was embarrassed when at the end of the play I was introduced as the author and there were a few laughs from the audience. However, I thought I became more generally accepted at school through writing this play.

There were times, though, when life was difficult and I was still ridiculed, and then I went through hell. The teachers stood back and allowed me to fight my own battles because they thought the label 'teacher's pet' might make matters worse. The school caretaker was a great ally and would often come to my rescue. He never said a word but his presence was enough to send my tormentors running. Many a time my coat would be thrown high over the bars in the cloakroom or up a tree in the school playground where it was impossible for me to get it down. On these occasions I was always relieved to see the caretaker appear to retrieve my coat when everyone had miraculously disappeared. It was as though he did not want anyone to see him helping me.

When my form did physical training I usually joined in and tried to play as the others did, but now we had a new teacher who asked me to sit and watch.

19

I hated this and felt different from the rest. Fortunately the headmaster saw me watching the others and wanted to know why. Obviously he had a word with the teacher and I was allowed to join in, although I didn't think I was popular with the physical-training teacher as a result. But I was still so scared of the other children.

I had an awkward streak and I wanted to try and feed myself. Mother said I was not ready for this. I made too much mess and took too long. However, my tantrums were such that she had to allow me to have my own way. Mother was constantly telling me not to suck my food but to chew it.

We had a large table in the centre of the living room which was used by everyone for all sorts of activities. We had the parlour too, but that was seldom heated and was kept for when we had visitors. The living room was always a centre of activity and the table was invariably being used for something or other. My father and I had the same old argument time after time. Each evening I practised my writing, using one hand, and my father counted the money he had taken that day, both of us using the table at the same time. In order to steady my hand while I was writing, I put a lot of pressure on pencil and the table shook as I wrote. Father's piles of coins were knocked over; he had to count them again and got annoyed. After this happened one evening, we all sat down to our meal. As often happened, my arm – the one used for feeding myself – went into a spasm. It sent the contents of my spoon across the table and they hit father in the face. He accepted this as an accident, but mother was not sure that I had not done it to get my own back for the quarrel father and I had earlier!

Gradually my writing was improving and I could write for short periods using one hand. I had made friends in school and although they didn't always understand my words, I was able to communicate with them by using speech and gesture. I had one special friend who also had a disability. This was Eileen. Many of the children gave her a bad time and she too was often laughed at; we found we had many difficulties in common. We were not included in the other children's activities away from school and we felt that others tended to get more pleasure out of life than we did. I had a pet mongrel, and I loved him but knew there should be something better. So Eileen and I made a plan.

My mother almost had a heart attack when I asked if I might go to the cinema alone. Until now I had always gone with one of my brothers. My going alone was a case for family discussion and for a start everyone wondered why I wanted to go. They are also concerned about how I would cope with a crowded bus and the busy town centre. I was not very steady on my feet and I could be easily knocked over. Sometimes if I fell, I still could not get up by myself. Actually, I had no intention of going on my own. I had arranged to go with Eileen, but I am not going to tell my family that, as they would not understand and probably not approve either.

My awkwardness and tantrums won the day as usual and I was given permission to go into town next Saturday.

The great day had arrived. I got on the bus at the stop at the bottom of the street and looked towards the next stop where Eileen should be waiting. The bus is full and I am afraid that Eileen would not be able to get on. Luckily she did. We had to stand all the way into town but I was quite safe as there was a pole to hang on to.

The town was very busy and I was a little scared. I did not want to hold on to Eileen's arm but neither did I like to be in a crowd when people were rushing about with their shopping bags. However, Eileen and I had no trouble in getting to the cinema and I felt quite grown-up as I paid for two tickets from the money I had saved from the jobs I did for father in the bakehouse.

When we got inside the cinema it was dark. Always before, one of my brothers had taken me by the arm as we looked for a seat but today I was not with a familiar guide. I did not expect to react to the darkness as I had. My balance had gone, I felt very frightened and the only thing I could do was drop to my knees and crawl. I felt embarrassed but Eileen said I worry too much and as it was a new experience, what did I expect?

We both enjoyed the film although my mind is leaping ahead and wondering if the lights will be on at the end. I did not fancy crawling out. I felt undignified enough crawling into darkness but the thought of crawling from the cinema was even worse. I need not have worried because when the lights did come on I was able to walk out normally.

Mother asked me all about my visit to the cinema and wanted to know if I met anyone I knew. Of course I answered with an emphatic 'no' but something in mother's smile made me feel uneasy... As I lay in bed later, Joe told me that he was assigned to follow me this afternoon to make sure no harm came to me and he saw me with Eileen. He gave me a lot of stick about it as though I was involved in a big love affair. Next, father and mother pulled my leg as I ate breakfast. I tried desperately to explain about Eileen but they only understood what they wanted to. Despite all the ribbing, the experience of going into town alone gave me confidence. Having had this experience, I wished to learn to dance with Eileen. There were a number of church halls around my home which have dances each Saturday evening, mostly attended by older women and children. Eileen and I thought it might be fun to go along and teach ourselves to dance. At first, mother would not hear of it. She said that I was too young at fourteen to be out dancing on Saturday evenings. However, Eileen's mother was going with us, so I was eventually allowed to go. Soon it became the usual practice for Eileen and me to go dancing every Saturday, although her mother did not often come with us. We got along very well together but I never had anything to eat or drink as it would have been too embarrassing in public. I was conscious that I did not chew my food. Mother was always on at me not to suck, but I could not chew. I was often sick after I had eaten and the doctor said it was because I bolted my food and should chew it more. I knew what he meant. I watched my family eat but when I tried to chew like they did, I found I could only suck. Still, I made less mess when I ate than I used to, so I must have been improving.

Eileen and I often laughed at and discussed the attitudes of people towards us at these evenings. They talked to us as though we were five-year-olds, they put on my coat and did up my buttons, and they helped us down the steps; older women had even been known to give up their seats to us. We had decided that the only way to stop this kind of thing is for us to act more like normal fourteen-year-olds. We decided to leave the dance early and wait in the cloakroom, ready to hold the coats for the older women; we were going to help them down the steps and if they spoke patronisingly, we were going to admire something about them. This was the night when we were to begin our new tactics and as I usually spoke only to my family and a very few friends, I felt dreadfully nervous. Here it came, a stroke on the cheek.

'Aye, he's a grand lad. Have you brought your little girlfriend for a dance? Aren't they lovely?' This is addressed half to Eileen and me and half to the company around us.

I replied, 'I do like your dress.'

Now the woman was asking those around her in a mystified voice, 'Did he try and talk to me?' Then Eileen is addressed. 'What's he saying, what's he saying? He did talk to me, didn't he?'

I want to run and hide, for now this woman was announcing to those within earshot, 'Aye, isn't he lovely, he tried to talk to me,' as though a miracle was happening. The opening notes of another dance allowed Eileen and me to escape but I felt depressed, even though Eileen was trying to talk me out of my gloom.

Eileen and I suffered great indignities from many people who misunderstood our friendship. They could not understand that Eileen and I had joined forces because it was an easy way out for us. We both felt a barrier between ourselves and 'normal' people, and we found a companionship in each other's company that is a substitute for the loneliness we knew we would both suffer if we had not befriended each other. We were brutally realistic and told each other frequently that we would not be such friends if it were not for our differences.

Many people of our age group had special relationships with one or several friends and discussed all kinds of problems which are part of the transition from childhood to adulthood. Many of these relationships hold something special, something that gives them strength and confidence, and, not least, a social life. Although Eileen and I had an excellent relationship, an element was missing, something that I could not put a name to but which is necessary to every close relationship. I was lonely and wished to be more popular and to have more friends. Although I welcomed Eileen's friendship, I was still frustrated when I failed to make friends with others. Fortunately I had a close relationship with my brothers and this was some compensation for the lack of outside friends. I envied the ease with which others seemed to form groups. It seemed to be such a difficult thing to do. It was not just a question of communication; I felt there were other elements involved. I wondered what skills I had not developed during my early isolation. I felt that others had an advantage over me inasmuch as they began to make friends at an early age while I was stuck in the house with my mother, unable to walk. I also thought of the years when I had to go to the girls' playground in school rather than the boys' playground, and wondered whether this was good for me. I didn't know whether I would have learned more about how to make friends in the boys' playground, but I seemed to be trying to figure out in my own mind how I could make friends and why I felt so awkward whenever I had the opportunity of integrating and getting to know more people. I had discussed this problem with my mother, who said that there were a great many people who found it hard to make friends, but this was of no solace to me. Eileen had the same problem and like me could not understand why, or find a solution.

At last I felt I may have found a relationship which may be of help to me. John had returned from military service had married and had a baby boy. I spent a great deal of time with this family and my nephew gave me something that was intangible and undefinable but which I knew I had never felt before. He always welcomed me and seemed to like having me around. He was actually demanding my attention and did not seem to tire of me. I loved the feeling this gave me. My brother and his wife were friendly and shared much of their life with me. My sister-in-law has a hearing problem and had been taught to lip-read, so she could tell what I said easily. These splendid people were my constant companions and offered me a relationship which is different from the others I have. When I speak to my sister-in-law, I felt like I'd been freed from a prison and from a darkness. I knew she must have got fed up with me because I talked to her non-stop. It was such a relief to speak to someone and be understood 100 per cent. Not only that, but having a two-way conversation is something which was new to me and it released a lot of my frustration. There were times when my brother was cross because I wanted to monopolise his wife's time but then he apologised and said he knew it was hard for me.

Obviously John needed time with his wife and family without me around and I was asked not to visit him on Sundays. After all, I was there almost every other day. I sometimes went straight from school and if his wife was at our home I offered to push the pram up the big hill to their home so that I could be with them for a little while.

By now my sister had also had a little boy and I was invited to tea with the family each Sunday. They didn't have a car so we went for walks or played Monopoly and my sister and I ended up giggling together. Harry had always been patient with me and tried to understand my speech. He also helped me to write using only one hand and told me I must try to form the letters more slowly and then my handwriting would improve. They had just bought their home and were decorating it. They hoped to make a garden in the backyard by taking up some of the paving stones. I wished to help and I offered to make the garden for them but Olive said the stones are too heavy and I may hurt myself. Harry thought I should try and do what I can, so here I was, breaking up paving stones and moving them to the bottom of the yard. As my sister said, they were heavy, but I was sure I could manage if I took my time. The garden was finished and Harry said my sister was really proud of it, more so than she would have been if he had done it.

The time was approaching when I had to leave school and there was much speculation about what I was going to do. Many people had ideas about what they thought I should do and I was feeling anxious. The majority of children at school had work to go to. Even Eileen had got a job as a clerk in the office of a coal merchant in Mincing Lane. Joe was a great consolation to me. He thought we should plan what I could do if I didn't get a job straight from school and he outlined all the jobs I could do in the bakehouse to help father. Father preferred that I find work elsewhere; he thought I would never ever be able to take over the bakehouse completely and that if I started working for him, the authorities may

24

not help me to find work and I might be worse off in the long run.

There was a sweetshop for sale near our house and father proposed to buy it for me so that I might make a living through it. He was prepared to mortgage the house and the bakehouse to buy it and grandmother was also willing to lend some money, but I didn't want the shop. People could not tell what I said and that would be a distinct disadvantage for a shopkeeper! Mother was also against the idea because she was concerned about all the debt we would incur in buying the shop. My sister-in-law discussed it with me and told father how I felt. He was keen to listen and when he fully understood my viewpoint he agreed with me. So the idea of the shop was out.

I was now the only one in my year at school without a job. I had seen many people about work but they were all discouraging. I went for a medical because I had to register as a disabled person and the doctor who saw me said that I was not really fit or capable for work and when I was eighteen I would receive an allowance of some kind for my support. I felt very depressed and cried myself to sleep each night. Joe comforted me when he heard my sobs and tried to cheer me. He was more hopeful than I was that a job would come along. He had been called into the army and I realised that this would never happen to me. I also started to wonder whether I should ever be married or even have a girlfriend. It was bad enough being the way I was, but not having a job made things worse... I could not see me being of any worth to anyone. Who would want to associate with me? My abilities were so limited. I felt so miserable and ill that I stayed in bed and refused to get up.

I had been in bed for about two weeks and the doctor said I should get up tomorrow. Mother was being very mischievous, and said she had a surprise for me but wouldn't tell me what it was until she heard me laugh again. It had to be something nice, for she had a gleam in her eye.

I had to be carried downstairs as I had grown so weak that I could not walk and this worried me, but the doctor said I would be all right in a few days. He told me I had lain in bed for too long and that the medicine he gave me had made my limbs too relaxed. I couldn't feed myself either but mother said I would be able to again in a little while. I felt sad and desperately wished I could get work, but now I couldn't walk anymore, my chances were even worse. I wondered if it was worth making the effort to try to walk or feed myself again. My family, not surprisingly, were fed up with me and said it was time I pulled myself together and got better. Father was threatening not to carry me down the stairs if I did not try to walk and mother said she would not feed me anymore, I had to feed myself. I hadn't eaten for two days and mother and father were arguing because father wanted to feed me but mother said if I was hungry I would feed myself. Mother was insistent and at last I tried. I thought there was more food down the front of me and on the table than I had managed to get in my mouth, but mother was pleased and had taken me on her lap to feed me my pudding. If I tried to walk to the front door and back, mother said she would tell me her secret. I had never wobbled so much in my life as I did when I walked down the lobby; I made it to the front door but I couldn't get back because my legs wouldn't go. Mother had to carry me back. I wondered if she would still tell me her secret.

My father arrived home from work as mother and I reached the top of the lobby. He wanted to know why mother was carrying me, and mother told him what happened. As she sat me in a chair, she was telling father that she had been to visit a man whom she used to know many years ago when she worked in the cotton mill. He was the cashier at a mill near to us and he said that if I could walk again, he would get me a job as a warehouse boy. This was mother's surprise. I couldn't believe it. Father wanted to know when this happened.

Mother said some time ago but she wanted to be sure that I was going to recover before she told me, as she thought it would have affected me badly if I knew I had a job but could never get to it. Now she was sure that I would get better. If only mother had told me before! I felt better already. The promise of a job was all I needed; I could feel determination return. I realised that my illness had been largely psychological.

The doctor was pessimistic. He agreed that my illness could have happened because I could not see any hope for my future, but he also said that according to medical facts I should not be able to walk at all and that maybe my walking days were over. But he was wrong before and I knew I should walk again. Walking did not hurt me but my legs felt heavy and dragging. Still, if I used the bakehouse each day to practise, I knew I would get better. After all, in the past, hadn't the doctor said I would improve? I wondered if he was doubting this now. I thought it was time that I knew what was really wrong with me but mother said she did not know and did not really want to know as she had every confidence in the doctor: he said I would grow out of it and even I had to admit that I had made physical progress. When I asked the doctor what had been wrong with me all my life he was evasive and told me that too much knowledge would be bad for me.

One of my teachers had come to visit me in my home and he offered to arrange for some of the boys in my year to push me to school in a wheelchair, but I refused. I had been away from school for five weeks and I would have liked to get back, but I preferred it if two boys were to come and help me walk to school. I had two friends coming for me on Monday morning and I would walk to school between them and lean on them if necessary. I learned to ignore the doctor. It was no use discussing my plans with too many people. They only understood a little of what I said and I felt more frustrated about this than previously. I still couldn't understand why people couldn't hear the words I spoke the way they sounded in my head.

I made it to school that morning and everyone seemed pleased to see me. I was glad to be back.

It was a little difficult to walk home at lunchtime but I managed with the help of my two friends. Mother was insisting that I go to bed to rest that afternoon and was going to see the headmaster to arrange for me to go to school for the morning session only until I got stronger.

I still had real difficulties in eating. I was so frustrated that around this time I would disappear at meal times and visit a neighbour Mrs Heap. This neighbour had been part of my life since my birth and I called her Mammy Heap. With wonderful patience Mammy Heap taught me how to use a knife and fork and I was able to cut up my own food. Mother was so annoyed and embarrassed because I had invited myself to someone else's home for meals but Mammy Heap really didn't mind and continued to work with me. I was really proud of the progress I had made and when my family saw me using a knife and fork I was hailed like an award winning Olympian!

It was four weeks to the day before I started work and I had to go and meet the manager of the mill. It was very noisy and I was alarmed at all the machinery but I was keen to work and the manager was prepared to employ me.

I liked the idea of starting work more and more and it was comforting to know that I had an aunt and uncle who worked at the same mill. Eileen's mother did too.

My walking improved and I felt as well as I did before I became ill. The doctor insisted that from now on I visit him once a week whether I was sick or not, and so the Wednesday evening visits began. I needed to be fit to start work and because I'm afraid of getting overtired I went to bed at 7:30 each evening. This made my family laugh but I was not taking any chances. I didn't want anything to stop me from starting my job after the New Year's holiday.

CHAPTER THREE

My fourteenth year was a difficult time for me; it was our last year at school and all the other students were looking forward to leaving school and getting a job. I was constantly told by more than one professional that I would never work. At this time I felt utterly rejected, not just by being told I would never work but also by the past bullying and harassment from my peers and the medical and educational authorities. I did not have too many friends and not knowing what the future held for me caused me to feel rather inadequate and terribly rejected. It was as though I'd lived most of my life under that awful feeling of rejection, not really understanding why. My family accepted me but outside of my family I felt rejected and that rejection made me feel a lesser person to others! I consider how rude and awkward I was to my family at this time. I don't think I felt sorry for myself, maybe I was angry but I remember feeling haunted by rejection and it made me Mr Nasty, not a very nice person around my family.

Of course my family did not reject me, they responded to my rages with an increase of love and support, actually ignoring what the professionals said, actually visiting factories, workshops and offices in the vicinity of our home, looking for work for me. Mum got me a job through her association with one of her work colleagues from when she worked in the mill! So two months after my fifteenth birthday I went to work in a cotton mill as a warehouse boy and with this job my mood changed and I was no longer Mr Nasty.

My duties were to bundle and stack the large and heavy bales of cloth after they had been inspected. This proved really difficult for me but within a very short time I developed the physical strength to throw these heavy bundles around as needed. Another aspect of the job was to carry messages from the staff of the warehouse to other departments of the mill. This was the most daunting aspect of the job for many reasons – in the weaving shed I had to walk through moving machinery, sometimes down a long alley about two feet wide with moving parts of machinery at each side of me. My walking and my balance weren't that good and it was so scary but I did it and improved from doing it. Whenever I entered the weaving shed it was to deliver a message to someone and the shed was extremely noisy! The weaving shed was a vast space which housed over a thousand looms, all weaving and adding to the tumultuous noisy environment. Each individual mechanical part of the machinery contributed to the mighty roar. One had to speak mouth to ear, literally mouth to ear. I had such a tiny and weak voice. Was it difficult!? For both parties it was difficult. But amazingly most weavers were really patient with me which made me relax. The more I relaxed, the better my speech became. Of course, most of the weavers were able to lip-read but my lip patterns were not easy to read. The older weavers were absolutely smashing to me – they actually corrected some of my immature and irrelevant behaviour. Many of them were not beyond giving me a clip round the ear. I learned social skills and acceptance. I learned quickly – some of the weavers administered a hefty wallop! Often I had to take messages to the 'men only' departments and they would tease and take the mickey. It made me revert back to former times when other children would make fun of me and be cruel, and my confidence would fail me. But then I witnessed how these 'men only' departments were with the other warehouse boys. There was no difference in how the men spoke to me and how they spoke to the other boys! There was a big difference in how I reacted! The other boys had experience of using verbal language; I had not. I had no rehearsal, no correction, no experience of verbal interchange. I had to learn. I think I learned more by observation than anything else. It also took confidence to answer back. The first time I did answer back very cheekily will always stick in my memory! My verbal opponent was gobsmacked, speechless, and the whole department 'roared' and applauded. I learned so much about myself as a warehouse boy and so much about the social aspects of life. During my school life I had been taught many negative lessons. Teachers would exclude me from activities, fail to correct my work and allow me to get away with things others didn't get away with. The fact that I was different was negatively reinforced throughout my school life but when I started work I had to conform! I was paid to do a job and no one else was going to do it for me. The message was clear: either conform and do the job or get out. The cotton mill was my finishing school and taught me more than ever my formal education did. I shall be ever grateful to the workers of the cotton mill, particularly my two fellow warehouse lads. The whole workforce accepted me and expected me to do my job. That expectation boasted my confidence, my self-value and my self-image. They shared and helped me to overcome my problems. I was taught how to behave, how to interact, positive skills and aspects which would normally be taken for granted.

Eileen had a wonderful singing voice and begun singing lessons. Her teacher was Miss Nuttall and because I was earning a wage I was able to pay for elocution lessons. I'm sure Miss Nuttall found it difficult to work with me but I gained a lot of knowledge from my elocution sessions which, with the help of Eileen and with constant practice, improved my speech considerably.

After three years as a warehouse boy I was promoted. I became a 'cut looker'. This involved inspecting rolls of material from the looms assigned to me. I would inspect the material, discuss any faults with the weaver and often involve others who were responsible for the mechanics of the particular loom involved in producing the faulty fabric. I was attending college towards gaining City and Guilds in textiles. So I knew the rudiments of weaving. Each time I called a weaver to see me in the warehouse, the weaver's looms would stop producing and the weaver would lose money. Weavers were paid for what they produced. Also, I had the power to reduce their pay for faults or shoddy work. None of the weavers liked to be called to the warehouse and most were aggressively protective and argumentative with me. I had neither the confidence nor the verbal skills to cope and maybe I took their bombastic torrents personally. This, linked with the poor quality of my social life, caused me great frustration and I found solace in alcohol. Eventually, I stopped drinking but the temptation and the urge has never left me. Maybe the addiction has lessened with the years but there are still fleeting moments when I long for the oblivion that I experienced from alcohol. But I never indulge; it's against my religion, I have a wife, family and grandchildren to consider and really if I can't be stronger than a bottle of alcohol, what kind of a human being am I?

Because of health-related problems, I had to leave the mill after working there for seven years. I claimed unemployment benefits and visited the 'dole office' every week. At the dole office, the staff were at a loss as to what to do with me and they introduced me to a disability rehabilitation officer who reinforced all the negatives from my childhood. He said I had to have a medical! The outcome of the medical was pretty dire and I demanded that most of the nonsense stated in the medical report be removed from my records. I pointed out that I had worked for seven years and it was now reported that I was unemployable! Eventually, I found my own job. I took a temporary job in London with a national charity as a kind of courier. My job was to meet foreign visitors to our country and guide them to establishments around our nation which catered for the needs of children and adults with disabilities. This took all my strength of will in developing my self-confidence to do the many varied demands of this job.

I saw an advertisement for it in the evening paper:

National charity require person to act as escort to foreign visitors investigating the English system of caring for disabled people. Training will be given for this temporary appointment.

I applied to a London post-office box number even though my mother and father didn't like the idea – I was fed up with sitting around with nothing to do but help in the bakehouse now and again.

I received a letter in the post calling me for an interview and giving me more details of the job. If I were lucky enough to be appointed, I would be living in a hotel in London during the weeks I was required to work.

Although it was an exciting prospect I didn't feel that I had the confidence necessary for such a job. Still, I would have to pluck up courage and travel to London, as I didn't have any other options. I explained all about myself when I applied for the job so the people who sent for me had some idea of the kind of person I am. I had been away from home on my own before. I was sent to an Employment Rehabilitation Unit in Leicester for six weeks by the dole office. I had also gone on holiday on my own to the Isle of Man. Surely if I can cope with going to the Isle of Man and Leicester on my own I can travel to London for an interview?

If I thought of how I might manage to do such a job I felt real panic so I couldn't allow my thoughts to go beyond the interview itself.

Others might make a little less of going for a meeting in London, but I had all kinds of fears. Not having been there before, I wondered how I would react to a busy city. What to do about food was another worry. As I would be travelling overnight, I did not like the idea of taking sandwiches. Since I might be away from home for twenty-four hours, I felt such snacks may not be adequate. The long train journey would add complications too; I found it difficult to eat and drink when I was motionless, so the jogging of the train could have been disastrous.

I decided to buy a new suit for the interview as I was sure my confidence would increase if I were looking the best I could. The cashier in the bank where I went to get money for my suit must have thought I was an idiot. I tried to sign the withdrawal form with a fountain pen, which was silly because I can write more easily with a biro. The ink would no flow so I shook it to try and get the ink to the nib; then it came out, all of it, a big blob on the floor of the bank.

'I am sorry, I have made a puddle on the floor. Do you have a mop please?' I asked the cashier.

'What do you mean, you have made a puddle on the floor?' asked the cashier, with her face registering absolute disgust.

'No, not that. All the ink has come out of my pen on to your floor and I would like something to clean it up with,' I explained. The relief on the cashier's face confirmed that she had thought that I had wetted the floor myself. I may have been oversensitive but once again I wondered if it was just my impeded speech (as well as my obvious physical difficulties) that led her to think that way. Or could it have been that I am, in a more complicated way, language-disabled, that I used the wrong word structure in my request? So much which naturally comes to most still seemed terribly and dauntingly sophisticated to me. When I spoke to people, I often found that I should have worded things differently, to make what I was saying clearer.

***

It was almost time for me to leave home to get the 9:30 overnight train to London. I did not know who was in a worse state, me or mother. If she knew how scared I really felt she would not have allowed me to go, but I was putting every effort into appearing calm and relaxed. Mother had a thousand don'ts for me: don't let people see your money, don't play cards on the train with strangers, don't go to sleep on the train without first making sure people cannot get at your money. It is impossible to remember all her don'ts and I think she was a little too fussy.

I had worked it all out. I got into Euston at 6:30am and I was going to get my breakfast in a café behind the station that Eileen told me about; then I would return to the station to change into my new suit and leave my case in the left-luggage office. After that I would have a little time to look around before my interview at ten o'clock.

I found the café Eileen told me about but I was not finding it easy to go inside. Being so early in the morning I thought it might be empty but I was wrong, it was full of people. I just didn't have the confidence to walk in and have breakfast. I walked around the block, hoping that the café would empty. It was silly. I was hungry and I had two options: either I stayed hungry or I could pluck up courage and walk into the café and order. There were tables free where I could sit on my own and there was a waitress, so I would not need to carry anything to my table. If I were to do anything embarrassing, it would not matter as no one knew me around here. After telling myself this I took a deep breath and walked in. I found a table in the corner and the waitress approached to take my order. I had to repeat myself for the fourth time as the waitress could not understand me but I could not allow that to bother me. All that mattered is that ultimately I had got breakfast.

What a feeling of achievement. I had travelled to London, ordered and eaten a meal in a public place and changed my clothes. Usually my mother had to help me to button my shirt neck and cuffs and sometimes to tie my shoelaces, but here I was looking quite smart and feeling comfortably fed – all through my own efforts.

The next step was to find a taxi and get to my interview. I hesitated for so long before I went into a café earlier that morning and it had taken me quite a while to dress myself, so nearly all the time had gone. It didn't matter, though. I could have a look around London after my interview.

Three other people were in the waiting room. I had problems with the receptionist on my way in as she thought I said my name was Thompson, but after I spelled it out for her she found it on the list. The waiting room was quiet and everyone looked tense. What chance had I? All of these people looked far more able than I felt I was and I could not understand why I had been called here against such odds. The longer I sat here, the less confident I felt.

The first woman to be called for her interview had just returned to the waiting room looking flushed. She was gathering up her things ready to leave. She was in the interview room just ten minutes and it seemed an age.

My name was called and I was shown into the interview room. There were two men and a woman waiting to see me. I felt ill at ease when I first entered the room, but these people were very nice and skilled in making people feel relaxed. As I answered their questions I remembered that I needed to make my voice come through the top of my head to give my speech more clarity. I answered many questions and discussed the problems that I might face while living away from home. I thought that I had spoken with a lot more confidence than I actually felt. I had been asked to take a seat in the waiting room as I may be needed again. I did not know what this meant; the woman who was just called in for an interview just before me was not asked to wait, so why was I?

Sitting there I had watched the third person leave and go home and now the fourth person returned and was also waiting. It was nerve-racking sitting there. It was quiet and time seemed to be passing so slowly. My stomach muscles were twitching violently. They always do when I am nervous but today I could see myself jerking around the middle of my body. We had been sitting there for about twenty minutes and I was beginning to think that we had been forgotten. The other man had been called in again and I was left alone in the room… That did not last long – the other man returned to the waiting room after only a few minutes and was preparing to leave the building. Now I was being called in once again.

'Come and sit down, Mr Counsell. We are sorry you have had such a long wait but these things take time, don't they?' said the woman as I enter.

I sat on the chair in front of the desk facing the three people who interviewed me earlier and tried to conceal my wriggling hand by hiding it between my crossed thighs.

'Well Mr Counsell, we have decided to offer you a position and would like you to begin next Monday,' said one of the men. The three of them rose from the chairs and offered their hands in congratulation.

I was stunned and speechless. I could not believe it. I knew I was being addressed but the words would not penetrate, I was so shocked.

Outside on the pavement I felt sick and I could feel my body trembling. I did not know whether this was because the interview was over or whether it was the realisation of what I'd let myself in for. My mind was in turmoil; I was to leave home and live in London and be trained for a job which would require me to meet strangers and take them around the country. I was going to need much more confidence than I felt at that moment. I was going to try very hard to make a success out of this extraordinary opportunity.

Wandering around London and looking at some of the places that had just been familiar names to me eased my tension a bit, and now I was feeling hungry again. If I was going to begin work in London I had better get used to being independent; I was not going to repeat my breakfast performance. The first café I saw I was going to walk into, no matter how crowded it was, and order a meal. If I could act with confidence then maybe I would appear more normal. I must have looked odd that morning as I walked around and around, continually coming back to look inside that café.

Somehow I was in Baker Street and there was a café down a side street. No uncertainty this time. I walked through the door and sat at a table. I was pleased: I did not look to see how many people were in before entering, nor did I look at the menu in the window. The waiter came for my order and rather than say it to him, I showed him the menu and pointed at what I would like to eat. It was much quicker to order this way than to try and get the waiter to understand my speech.

Today had been one of the best in my life for increasing my confidence. It could be the start of something new. I did not know how I was going to cope with foreign visitors nor how I was going to manage living away from home in London, but other people had shown their faith in me and I would do my best. Doubts and inadequacies had to be hidden.

Looking round London was fun and I hoped that while I worked here in the next few months, I could visit many more sights. All the time I kept thinking how truly amazing it was that I had done so much that day without real embarrassment or hitch. I was even more amazed that I had been appointed to such an attractive and demanding job.

***

Miss Partridge, one of the people who interviewed me, was at the station to meet me. She took me to my hotel. My bedroom was on the first floor and was really quite ordinary; it contained a bed, a chair, a chest of drawers and a wardrobe. We arrived there about five o'clock and as dinner was not until 6:30 I had time to change and settle in.

The nearer dinnertime got, the more nervous I began to feel about going down to the dining room. I would be all right if I had a table on my own but I did not think I could share a table with others.

There really was no need for me to worry, for I had my own table in the dining room and I felt silly for having caused myself such ferment in thinking about this meal. One of the other tables was occupied by a young man who was also dining alone. It would be good practice for me if I could get into conversation with him. My table was between this young man's and the door so that he had to pass me to leave the dining room. I decided to wait at my table until he finished his meal and left the dining room. As he walked past me I rose and said to him, 'That was a nice meal.'

'Yes, the hotel food is quite good. Are you on holiday?'

'No, I have come to work in London. Have you been here long?'

'No. Like you I am working here for a short time.' We left the dining room and stood in the hotel foyer.

'I have arrived only today. I don't know London, as I have never been here before. I am staying here at the hotel for a while. What is there to do in the evening?'

'Nothing much in the hotel. I have been here a week. I would be glad to show you around the district a little if you would like that.'

'That is kind of you. I would enjoy that.' We exchanged names and arranged to meet again in the lobby in ten minutes.

***

I learned from our brief association that evening that Tim is a little older than I am. He had a mop of black hair and he came from Bradford. He took me all round the district and seemed to accept me very well. When we parted late that evening it was as though we had been friends for years. It was a marvel to me that I could leave home this morning, settle into a new situation and make a friend so quickly. The shame was that I could not share the excitement I felt. I was not sure that anyone could possibly understand what it had been like for me to be released from the bonds of almost complete non-communication to this sort of freedom and the stimulation of being understood, even by strangers.

I went to sleep thinking that tomorrow might be the first day of a new life, for having met Tim and talked with him without too many misunderstandings or problems gave me huge confidence at just the right time. I knew that my job was going to offer me an opportunity to grow and build on my potential as never before.

Going down to breakfast that morning was not the ordeal that dinner was yesterday. I was no longer apprehensive or worried about the dining room. There were not many people having breakfast. It was a little early but I was keen to get to work. Tim was approaching my table.

'Good morning, Alan. Did you sleep well?'

'Good morning, Tim. Yes, thank you. Did you?'

'Yes. Do you mind if I join you? There is no need for us to sit separately.'

I felt panic rise as I wondered how Tim was going to take my style of eating. Because of my shaky hands, instead of raising the food to my mouth I had to bring my mouth down to meet my hand; my chewing process was unusual too, but I could not say no to Tim. That would be most impolite. I had to be sociable; it was part of my new self.

'Yes, Tim, please do join me.'

If only my family could have seen me. What would they have said? All the fuss they made about me coming to London, and not only have I made a friend, but Tim was actually asking me if I would like to go with him to the theatre tonight. He was seeking my companionship. What a thrill that was. Tim was a complete stranger yesterday and he couldn't have found it too embarrassing to talk to me otherwise he wouldn't have invited me to go out with him that evening.

Miss Partridge was waiting for me as I arrived early at the office and we got down to work straightaway. I had less than three weeks to find out all I could about the many associations that care for disabled people and I had to make arrangements for a number of visitors who would be coming to England in the next few months. I had lots of reading to do and many letters to send out about forthcoming visitors. I had the help of a secretary called Helen, and I learned more from her than from anyone else. She organised me, made all my appointments and advised me on the layout and structure of my letters. If it were not for Helen I think I would have made a shambles of the administrative side of my job.

One of my concerns, as always, was my style of eating. I would have to entertain overseas visitors and I was worried about my physical appearance at mealtimes. At the end of my first week I approached Miss Partridge about this. She had been friendly and helpful throughout my first week and she now invited me to lunch. We went to a restaurant which was rather classy and I was a little confused by all the elegance. However, I remembered being taught to start at the outside with the cutlery and work towards the plate. I even managed a glass of wine without too much difficulty. I received nothing but praise from Miss Partridge at the end of the meal.

'I think you got that meal out of me under false pretences, Alan. Your eating is quite acceptable, like everything else you do. You have no need to be concerned. Look, there is no mess and I didn't help you at all. Anyone who knew your difficulties would admire the way in which you cope. You have been watched closely all this week at the office and everyone is impressed. We are convinced that we got the right man for the job. So don't think too much about what you call problems; we are happy to have you with us and we like you just the way you are.'

I didn't know how to respond to such a speech, for I was embarrassed, but it was good to know that my employers approved of me.

Tim and I were dining out tonight. We fancied a change from the hotel. We had a drink in the bar before we left the hotel. This evening it was my treat and while I could not afford anything grand I wished to go to a restaurant which has a bit of style. Since I was in charge this evening, I acted with confidence but as I was speaking to the waiter to order the food, he put his ear down on a level with my mouth. This looked most peculiar but maybe he was having difficulty in understanding what I was saying and was trying to listen to me more closely. I was wrong. He stopped me in mid-sentence and said, 'You're drunk. I am sorry, we cannot serve you.'

Tim and I looked at each other in disbelief, for we had only had one drink. Tim was more shocked than I was.

'I am sorry, sir, I am not drunk. I do have a speech impediment and I have had just one drink, but I am certainly not drunk,' I reply.

'I cannot serve you. Kindly leave.'

Tim looked most embarrassed and the other diners were able to hear the waiter's accusations.

'You have made a mistake. You are quite wrong, my friend and I are not drunk and we would like to order a meal.'

'No, sir, he is drunk. We do not serve drunks in here. Would you kindly leave the restaurant?'

We could have argued forever but it was better that we left. We found another restaurant further along the road and we were served with our meal without any trouble. Tim was horrified about the incident in the first restaurant. I related a few more incidents from my past and I proved my point when we left the restaurant, by ringing for a taxi from a phone box. Five minutes after I had ordered the cab, Tim was ringing the same taxi firm to order one in his name. I knew that the car which I had ordered would not arrive. Sure enough, Tim's was here. Tim asked the driver to wait and rang to ask what happened to the taxi that I ordered.

'No taxi booked in the name of Counsell.'

'But I stood here with him and heard him book it.'

'I remember some drunk ringing in just before you rang but we never send a taxi if we know the customer is drunk.'

Tim and I had a much closer relationship after these two incidents and now that we knew each other better I told him some of the feelings I had before my first meal in the hotel. Tim could understand how I felt and see why my confidence was sometimes shaky, after seeing the two episodes tonight but he said that he was amazed at the way I managed.

I often look back on this period of my life and wonder how I did it. The fact is: I did it! My base was in London and so I often had to stay in accommodation, away from home. I would imagine my parents went through trauma whilst I travelled the country doing this job. They both expressed concerns before I even applied for the job. I had to take the job. I just could not sit around doing nothing anymore. The job was demanding and threw up lots of problems but it taught me how to manage myself and my own problems. It taught me how to put other people at ease. It taught me that I had a responsibility in relationships inasmuch as I had to meet people halfway and allow them to get used to my speech, my appearance, etc. I learned coping skills and I overcame fear as I met people and used the telephone to arrange hotel accommodation and travel for the visitors. I developed so much confidence from this time in my life.

It took a great deal of courage to leave home, even for a short period, and I think I learned that I had to forget all the rejection of my past and simply 'go for it'. I realised that fear would hold me back and I think my greatest fear was rejection and ridicule. I needed courage to allow myself to develop. Fear actually made me shrivel but courage allowed me to experience new things and to learn who I was and what I was. Courage helped me to set goals and to achieve!

After realising the power of courage and after working in London for just over a year, I applied to become a student nurse at a psychiatric hospital on the outskirts of Blackburn. I never thought I would be accepted. I applied thinking, 'nothing ventured – nothing gained'. To my absolute astonishment, I was accepted and I began an ongoing battle with older members of staff who were used to seeing the likes of me as patients rather than colleagues. I now had the confidence to retaliate. I became notorious for challenging. I challenged negative and disparaging remarks directed at myself and I challenged the management and treatment of some of the patients. I was so aware of my own experience of being threatened by the label of 'mental defective' that the phrase and notion of 'there but for the grace of God go I' struck chords of strong empathy in me and I really felt strongly about some of the practices I witnessed. The Medical Director of the hospital and the Chief Male Nurse, along with the Nursing Tutor, were very supportive of all my challenging and spent much time discussing issues with me, also helping me to understand the history and traditions of the hospital whilst encouraging me to continue to question and challenge.

Things became very difficult for me as a third year student nurse. I was supposed to learn how to give injections and measure and mix medicine and I knew that because of my shaky dexterity I would not be able to manage. I felt

I'd have to give up nursing and I was rather angry at this, for I thought it would confirm many of the negatives I had challenged in the older and more established nursing staff. When I discussed my intentions and my feelings with the Medical Director he offered me a job as the hospital's Welfare Officer. I attended Manchester University and gained my Social Work Qualification. This, together with the studies I did as a student nurse, also qualified me as a Mental Health Officer. I also gained qualifications in counselling!

I continued to work as the Welfare Officer but at this time, the sixties, the field of mental health rapidly changed because of the 1959 Mental Health Act. I found myself in charge of a rehabilitation unit with a great responsibility to prepare patients to leave this long-stay hospital. They had to be trained to live in appropriate accommodation, determined by their ability and by the local authority in which they lived before they entered the hospital. Some patients had to be found employment in the area of their new home and be trained to do that work. Many of the patients were classified as psychopaths and had been sent to hospital by the courts. These patients caused lots of complicated liaisons with various authorities and a few were transferred from hospital to prison. As I contacted and interacted with the many agencies and authorities concerned with the future placements of patients, I was often faced with rudeness and prejudice. Professional people who had not encountered the likes of me in responsible positions! Professional people who tried to ignore me and preferred to speak to others whom I managed rather than to me! Professional people who thought they were superior to me because they were able to 'speak properly'! Professional people, the likes of which had caused me and my family trauma and heartache in my early life! I became very assertive, if not aggressive, and I had to conquer and be an advocate on behalf of the patients I represented. My attitude had a positive affect on the staff of the rehabilitation unit I managed: they wouldn't dare treat a patient as anything else but their equal – their past training had taught them to take charge and to have power over the patients. Their past experience had been to work for the establishment; now I demanded that they worked with and for each individual patient. There were no rotas or set duties. We were a patient-oriented unit!

Eventually, I left the hospital service and trained as a teacher. I actually became a student at Cambridge University!

My teaching career was really successful in terms of rising to the status of senior positions rather quickly, which provided my family with a really good living and in terms of establishing my own philosophy. My first teaching post was at a boarding school for pupils who had physical and learning difficulties.

I taught the 15 plus-aged students. I'm afraid I rocked the establishment by refusing to teach the three Rs and other subjects on the curriculum. My class had been in education for at least the last ten years of their life and they were still being taught to read and write, etc. After all this time in education, none of them were able to read or write, therefore they had been taught to fail. I needed my students to succeed. They needed to succeed. So my timetable abolished most of the traditional subjects on the curriculum. We learned how to pair socks, how and where to put our clothes away. We learned where and how our clothes were washed and some of us learned to iron and press our clothes. Previously all these chores were done for them and had been done for them all of their lives. Most of my students didn't know what a washing machine was or did, as with an iron and other everyday appliances. We had a very practically oriented timetable. We went horse riding with the local Riding for the Disabled group. We went to the local leisure centre, we learned to swim and we practised archery. We went to the local mainstream school and joined in drama, art, woodwork and cookery lessons. We organised school trips and went camping and on long boats, etc. Three significant things happened. All the parents of my students said their sons and daughters had much more to talk about when they rang. The house parents reported that members of my class were happier, easier to cope with before and after school and wanted to help around the living quarters of the school. And the members of my class demonstrated much more confidence in many areas of their lives. They were experiencing success and sincere praise.

Because I took my students out and about and on residential trips, I needed to become qualified in first aid. I had to attend several centres before I found an instructor who would accept me. All said I would not manage the course because I had physical disabilities. I eventually met a female instructor who accepted me and at the end of a ten-week course I succeeded in obtaining a certificate in first aid!

Although the principal of the school was not at all happy with my curriculum and my style of teaching, he witnessed the success element and found it difficult to argue with my methods.

Fortunately for me, the principle left after my second term and was replaced by a man who encouraged and supported all my work and very soon I was promoted to House Master, a very senior position. With this new position came responsibility and new opportunities. One of those opportunities was to speak to various groups outside of school. My reputation grew and I was invited to speak to student teachers attending Cambridge University. For six years I was invited twice a year to speak about my educational philosophy and practise in special education. I had to pinch myself on more than one occasion. Me, who struggled so much with speech in my younger years and who people had such low expectations of. Was I really lecturing at Cambridge University? How I appreciated the power of speech, and still do today! What a thrill! An absolute blast to stand before any audience and speak, knowing that my speech is understood by all who hear my voice.

Many members of staff who worked at the boarding school were also resident within the grounds of the school and so it was very convenient for me to organise a school pantomime. At the end of the Christmas term every year throughout my employment, the staff entertained the students. I wrote, produced and directed this show! The rehearsals and all the organising had a profound effect on the staff; we got to know each other and became a better team.

I am the first to admit that I really cannot sing! I'd like to. I'd love to have a singing voice like my dad and my brothers but I have to admit, I do not really have a singing voice! However, after each pantomime, all who were involved in it were invited to a post-production party and one year I promised I would sing my favourite number at the party.

All were gathered and the anticipation and maybe the concerned respect caused the room to go completely silent. I appeared on the stage, acted very nervously, took some deep breaths, made it look as though I was trying to calm myself and nodded to my pianist who played the most complicated and elaborate introduction ever played. At the time I was supposed to sing I faked a fit of coughing and it took all my willpower for me not to laugh as I saw the concerned looks on the faces of my audiences.

Once again my pianist played the introduction at the end of which I sang, in my own unique way – forty four. I then bowed and walked from the stage. I had fulfilled my promise! I had promised to sing my favourite number. My favourite number happens to be 44!

Kathleen, my wife, is an accomplished pianist and the theory of music was a compulsory subject of my teacher training course. Whilst living at the boarding school, Kathleen and I formed a mixed choir. Kathleen played the piano and I directed. It was a lovely thing to be involved in and I learned how difficult it is to organise people who work on different rotas. I had to be really organised. But to be involved in directing this choir brought me so much pleasure and compensated for my lack of ability to sing!

My time at the boarding school lasted eight years. I was offered a senior post at another school, this time for students with just physical disabilities.

The pupils at this new school were quite different to my previous school inasmuch as they did not have learning difficulties. In my opinion, I would suggest that education had not really been a priority for the majority of them. Medical intervention was a major interruption to many of the students' education. Occupational, physio- and speech therapy appeared to be much more important than academia! Most of the students in my class had also spent a lot of time away from school in hospital having surgery, receiving treatment or convalescing! It was a major concern to me that no matter what lesson or educational programme I was involved in, with any individual or group, it was inevitably invaded by a therapist.

Students' ages in my class ranged from 14-16 and my philosophy was more social education, in the natural and real world, than classroom based. I still taught the three Rs but in a more practical way than normal.

I enjoyed real good relationships with the parents of my students and many confided in me.

One student had epilepsy. He had at least three or four fits a week and was on medication which zombified him. One day whilst talking to his parents who were worn out and anxious about dealing with their son's fits, I mentioned the Centre for Epilepsy at Chalfont St Peter in Buckinghamshire. I thought that by contacting them, the parents might get some support and might meet other parents with similar problems.

The parents duly made contact and the centre requested that their son become a resident at the centre for at least three weeks. At the end of that period the parents were told that their son's epilepsy was caused by food intolerances and if he followed a strict diet he would not need medication. This young man returned to school after having almost a full term away to adjust to living without the drugs he had taken for most of his life and he was unrecognisable. He was wide awake, full of energy and interested in all activities!

Of course, I had failure as a teacher. I continued to take pupils on school expeditions. One was on long boats. One of the students was 17 years of age and he could read well. I was working on his comprehension. He could read but did not understand the meaning of what he read. He was on the trip to become much more independent too.

He came to me on the first day of our trip and said he had an ear infection and had brought drops with him. I told him he could put his own drops in. 'Just read the label on the bottle!'

That evening, as all were getting ready for bed, I found this 17-year-old in a very unusual contorted position. I bellowed down the long boat, 'What are you doing?'

'Putting my ear drops in!' came the reply.

'Your ears are on your head, not your backside.'

'You told me to read the label and I'm only doing what it says.'

I grabbed the bottle from him and on the label was written: '1 drop in R ear.'

I wasn't wrong. His comprehension needed working on.

Even I never learn! This same lad was asked to mix four packets of instant whip. I explained that we had four boats in our fleet and there was one packet of instant whip for each boat.

'Read the packet and come back and tell me what you have to do and how you are going to do it,' I instructed as I steered the boat.

He reported back after a few minutes and explained he was going to put a pint of milk in a bowl, pour the powder onto the milk and whisk.

'That's really good,' said I. 'Well done! Put it in the fridge when you've finished and don't forget one packet for each boat!'

On retrieving the instant whip from the fridge for dinner, we found concrete! The lad had mixed all four packets in one pint of milk!

Will I ever learn?

After a few years I was given another promotion and part of my job was to work with and teach students with a short life expectancy. The school had an 'open door' policy, which meant that parents could walk into school at any time and talk with the staff, observe their child in school or ask questions. The parents got to know me and I got to know them and many of them had enough confidence in me to tell me what it was really like to live with a child who was going to die in the near future. I attended many funerals and some parents continued to visit me even after their child had departed this life. I had one mum who came to see me on a regular basis. Often she would tell me about her husband, who walked out on her almost monthly. He would come home from work, have a rant, as his wife called it, pack his bags and go. He always returned within a week but during the few days he was gone the wife found it extremely difficult. This couple had four children and the fourteen-year-old boy was a wheel chair user; he looked grossly overweight because of wasting muscles which was one aspect of his diagnosis – he was really heavy to lift to

45

the toilet, etc., and he was said to have less than a year to live.

I invited the dad to come and see me. He couldn't come to see me until after he had finished work. The first meeting was in the evening and he was very aggressive towards me. When I first met him he was very reticent and I could tell he was thinking, 'are you just another professional or do-gooder?' He had so many people from so many agencies prying into his life and making judgements – he had really had enough. I explained that I had no idea what it was like to walk in his shoes and I had no advice to give him. I told him that I thought his anger and aggression were justified and in his position I think my anger and aggression would be worse than his. During the conversation which ensured I was able to invite discussion, as sensitively as I could, about the fact that his son was very upset when he walked out on the family and I was concerned and wanted to know if there was any way I could help. After much discussion he agreed that he would not walk out on his wife anymore but he would instead come and talk to me. This father never left home again but came to visit me; more often than not he would appear just after the end of the school day, sometimes he would request to see me in the evening. I felt so sorry for him; it was so difficult for him. He loved his son so much and he had always had a vision and expectations for his family's future, including his son's. Now he was waiting for his son to die. He was contemplating all kind of things. How does one prepare for their son's death? He would ask questions to which I had no answers. He would blame himself, his genes and his ancestors. He blamed God. He would shout and swear. I provided cushions for him to throw and then he would cry. His sobs were awful and sometimes I would cry with him. The morning after each visit I would receive a thankful note from him which would tell me how great I was. I didn't feel great. I felt very useless. I mainly sat there listening to him and tried to look interested and intelligent. I also had six other sets of parents with the same issues. Many of them had social workers to support them but this particular family had been left without any support because of father's attitude and although the school, the school doctor and the education authority tried to get the much needed support, none materialised because dad had already told all the agencies he didn't want them involved.

At this time in my life my wife and I were really concerned about our youngest daughter. She was being bullied at school and was so unhappy. I did everything I could to stop this. I talked with my daughter and discussed strategies for her. I visited her school and spoke with her head of year. I spoke with the bully's father who laughed at me. I even spoke with the bully's grandparents, whom I knew, who said their granddaughter, the bully, was totally out of control and they were afraid of her and could not help. I even spoke to the bully herself who denied everything, said my daughter was lying, accused me of trying to get her in trouble with her father and laughed in my face.

I can't explain how I felt! I did not want to go to work. Each night as I was drifting off to sleep, in my mind I would hear the father of the dying 14-year-old shouting and swearing at me or I would see my younger daughter lying bruised and battered at the bottom of a long staircase after being battered and thrown down the stairs by bullies. I would eventually go to sleep but wake up feeling tired and bad tempered. It was not like the usual me. By the time I'd got ready for work I was exhausted. I didn't want to drive my car. I really had a crisis of confidence!

My wife insisted that I go and see our family doctor, with whom I got on really well. So insistent was my wife that she rang to make the appointment for me. As I entered the doctor's consulting room, I felt awkward. I didn't know how to explain how I felt. He just sat there and looked at me and said 'Well?' I think I shrugged my shoulders and he said, 'You look tired. Tell me what's up?' I mumbled and hesitated and tried to explain things.

Out of my confused mumblings came a conveyance of the basic rudiments of the miserable feeling I had. I said, 'I feel I want to give up – I just cannot go on. I used to be able to switch off and leave my work at work but now it's on my mind the whole time. I can't switch off. I feel tired. Not the kind of tired I usually feel at the end of the day but a heavy and exhausted tiredness which is not relieved by sleep.'

The doctor questioned me, told me I had to take at least a month off work and gave me tablets. I could not believe it. I hadn't had a day off work sick for twelve years!

The tablets he gave me had a horrible effect on me. They made me so dopey! Each time I sat down I would fall asleep. Everyone said I needed time to get used to the tablets but I felt and performed like a zombie. After three days I stopped taking the tablets.

At that time my elder daughter, who was in further education but had a part time job, brought a dog home from her work. The dog had belonged to the grandmother of one of her colleagues from work. The grandmother had died and none of her family wanted the dog, so it was doomed to be put down. My daughter, being rather sensitive and soft-hearted, could not bear to see a healthy dog put down. And so we acquired a dog which became a family pet, and I began taking the dog for walks.

The walks got longer and more strenuous daily. I would sit in the woods or by a woodland stream or in a deserted meadow and I would talk to my sometimes sleeping dog and if he wasn't sleeping; he would lick my hand or snuggle his chin in my lap as though he understood and was trying to show sympathy. Once I talked to my dog about my daughter being bullied and I began to shed tears. The dog actually licked the tears from my face. How come I could solve the problems of others but not help my own daughter?

This was a big issue and I could not resolve it. But how grateful I was for speech! Being able to verbalise one's thoughts, even to a dog, was kind of liberating. I wonder if, had I been able to talk to my parents, family or potential friends when I was younger, my problems and challenges would have been confronted better and the effects lessened inasmuch as I might not have internalised so many negatives. Maybe having the ability to verbalise my thoughts and feelings would have lessened the impact and the damage of those traumatic episodes in my life.

I was very aware of how my teenage children talked with their friends. They talked on the telephone for hours, much to my annoyance! They went out with their friends in the evening and a group of six or seven of them would end their evening together, gathered by the street lamp near our home, with a bag of chips each, purchased from a local chip shop, and they would talk! I am sure that talking with their friends and their peers helped them solve problems, helped them to reason things out. Helped them make sense of the world and aided their development. I never had that opportunity. Friends in my early teenage years just did not exist because my speech was so bad – no one, other than my immediate family, could understand a word I said. In my late teens, any friendships I might have formed were jeopardised by my cravings for alcohol. So maybe my development may have been restricted because of my communication problems!

However, being home from work and having 'sick notes' each week from my doctor was alien to me! Eventually, I was told by my G.P. that I was suffering from professional burnout and that, in his opinion, I should not return to teaching. What a blow. Absolute devastation! I had a mortgage. I had two teenage daughters in education. Where was I going to get work in the future? How was I going to support my family?

48

CHAPTER FOUR

I suppose I'd been away from work for a month when I was approached by a woman who wanted me to help with her 17-year-old son Adam. He had 'mild cerebral palsy' and a learning difficulty. I was initially reluctant to get involved but relented and went to meet this young man. He lived on a council estate and had been the victim of name calling and 'missile' throwing from a group of young people who also lived on the estate. These incidents had been dealt with by the police and by Adam's parents speaking with the parents of the culprits. The council estate had a good reputation in the area for having an excellent community spirit and the local press often reported acts of community-spirited humanitarian events where neighbourhoods helped each other or a family in dire distress! I do wonder if the anti-social activity aimed at Adam might have been caused by the mystique of the yellow bus which in previous years had picked Adam up every morning of his school life to transport him to the special school which he had attended, or the unexplained segregation from the other children as they all walked to local schools both as young children and as senior children. Adam's experience of anti-social behaviour had affected what little confidence he had and had added to his already low self-esteem and morale. I suspect his parents had asked me for help in desperation. A fellow member of the church I attended had spoken to the parents of my work with disabled children.

Adam had sparkling blue eyes and curly brown hair along with a cheeky, mischievous smile which made him appear attractive. He walked with a slight limp and his right hand felt clumsy as we shook hands when we met. He had left school at 16. On leaving school he had attended a Continuing Education Course at the local college but after attending for two weeks had refused to go because he didn't enjoy it and didn't like the other students. He then went to a Training Centre run by Social Services but he found it boring and refused to go. Mum was fed up with him hanging around the house and watching television all day. It became obvious that he couldn't read or write. He had indeed a learning difficulty around academia but this guy had a personality. He was really sociable and made conversation with me easily. He asked questions and was interested in people. He wanted to work and earn money. I hadn't a clue as to how I was going to help him. I had a friend who managed a leisure centre and to get Adam out of the house I introduced him to my friend and the gym. It was so difficult to get Adam to leave the house and I may have used bullying tactics disguised as psychology to get him to the gym in the first place. Once I got him there Adam showed a reluctance to use any of the apparatus and equipment at the gym, although in my opinion he had the physical ability to cycle, row and engage in many of the other activities. He constantly said, 'I can't do that!' However, after the first visit he did want to return and within a few days he was attending on his own. The staff were very persuasive and encouraged and cajoled until Adam could use all the gym equipment. He developed a rapport with the staff and over time Adam loved attending the gym. He would spend hours each day using the various apparatus and chatting to the staff. He became popular with many who used the gym and this social aspect alone increased his confidence.

The way he entered into banter with other people at the gym was remarkable. He had a very engaging way and a good sense of humour. His innocence gave him a unique attraction. His learning difficulty was a little obvious in a social setting. I witnessed that he had the ability to laugh at himself when his physical clumsiness caused any problems. As I witnessed him at the gym and received feedback from my friend, the manager, I became aware of a person rather than a set of problems. His parents had often said he was lazy. He wouldn't help around the house or the garden. I discovered his parents were rather negative about him and to him. They never gave him any praise and always criticised and tried to improve whatever task he undertook.

Quite a change came over Adam from attending the gym. He was experiencing success and he was receiving praise. I think too that he felt accepted by people at the gym and his confidence improved. Before this time, I think Adam visualised himself as a failure. I cashed in on his new found confidence and on his success at the gym and suggested we should look for a job for him. Father thought that the local supermarket might take Adam as one of the boys who collected trolleys from the car park. I knew I somehow had to stop his dad from reinforcing negatives. That proved to be very difficult!

I took Adam to the local Job Centre. They were worse than useless. It was obvious to me that Adam did not want to be with other disabled people. The staff at the Job Centre offered Adam courses and placements with other people with a learning difficulty. Adam's parents wanted Adam to take what was offered, and to say there was friction and quarrels in the family is an understatement. I wasn't sure that Adam's parents were aware of how Adam reacted in a social setting. So I suggested dad come and watch Adam at the gym! Within two hours dad had got the message. He said, 'I've never seen him like that before! He fits in well with that crowd! He holds his own!' Father was very quiet as I drove him home – rather thoughtful.

'Have you any idea what we can do with him?' Adam's father asked of me as we pulled up outside his home after our journey from the gym. Well, really, I hadn't. I needed to get to know Adam much more before I could give any advice or opinion.   But I did know we had to stop all the negatives and try to change Adam's image of himself from a can't do image to a can do or at least I can try image.

I had known Adam about two months when he celebrated his eighteenth birthday! On the occasion of his party he talked to me about his interest in cars. He had never mentioned this interest before and he invited me to take my car round to him the next day so he could wash it for me. What a dilemma! Could I trust him with my car? It would only need him to drop a cleaning cloth and pick up stones or grit and he would scratch my paint work. After all, his right hand was rather clumsy! I had to do a complete overhaul of my attitudes. I knew what it was like to have people make assumptions and to show a lack of confidence in me and here I was doing the same to others. I was so unaware of my own attitudes. I decided I must allow Adam to clean my car and left it with him for the morning.

I was amazed at the good job he did. My car shone like new, inside and out. I thought someone must have helped him, but he had done it all alone. Having seen the results of his handiwork, I contemplated if he could perhaps offer car washing as a business and at least contribute towards his keep at home. Without mentioning what was on my mind, I began assessing him in my own way. I asked if he would go shopping for me and if he would get me six items without giving him a list. He couldn't read a list anyway but he remembered all that I wanted. I asked if he would visit me at my home eight days ahead and told his family not to remind him. Through these kinds of activities I discovered he had an excellent memory.

Bill, a friend of mine who was a retired ex-police driver, assessed whether Adam would be able to drive. No problems there either.

When I explained to my friendly ex-policeman what I had in mind he offered to help in any way he could. After about a month of observing Adam in all kinds of 'set ups', I decided to discuss the idea of Adam washing cars for a living with his parents. They were so negative and full of 'what ifs'. I was able to answer all their negatives and I got them on my side. For this venture to work, I needed their co-operation and I needed them to be positive.

When the plan was explained to Adam his chest swelled and his face beamed at me. He was enthusiastic and eager. We needed money to set Adam up in business. I rang Bill. Bill and I met to discuss what was needed and how much we needed. When it came to driving lessons on our list, Bill crossed this item off, saying he would teach Adam to drive. It seemed to me that Bill was as enthusiastic as anyone about this project. After all, he confessed, he was at home with little to do other than take orders from his wife and look forward to a bowling match twice a week.

Adam's father had served in the Army when he was younger and one of Adam's older brothers was currently serving in the army and hadn't long returned from the aftermath of the Falklands war! I wrote a letter to the Royal British Legion and explained the situation and the proposal. They wanted to be involved but needed Adam's father's service number. Words cannot describe the frantic search of both dad's memory and the loft for this number. A great deal depended on finding this number. The number could not be found and into the gloom Adam suggested we call his grandma. Father's mother; she had the number and so The British Legion became involved. It was amazing! Suddenly we had all the money we needed to set Adam up in business. Bill bought an automatic car on Adam's behalf and began to teach Adam to drive. These driving lessons did not go smoothly but Bill was so patient and he persevered.

A change had come over Adam; he was much more responsible and responsive and – mother said – much easier to manage at home. Let me tell you, a change had come over Adam's parents as well. They were much more patient and kinder to Adam – much more supportive and positive. After all, maybe for the first time in the life of their son, they were experiencing hope and someone believed in him!

The man from The British Legion was so helpful, helpful beyond the call of duty. He spotted a yard, not five minutes' walk from Adams home. He contacted the owner of this yard and negotiated for Adam to use it free of any rent for a year.

The yard was at least half an acre and had a large shed with water and electricity. I don't know who was the more excited: Adam, his parents, Bill or the man from the Legion.

I had empathy with his parents. I knew they had heard lots of negatives about their son in the past. Everyone had very low expectations for Adam up until this point in his life.

His parents and I stood in their kitchen discussing Adam's future with great expectations and positivity. I got mum and dad to give a raspberry for everyone from their past who had been negative about Adam. Doctors, social workers, teachers, career guidance people; even educational psychologists were all given raspberries. I was kind of hoping that by blowing raspberries they were releasing negatives from their systems. It was a good exercise and the parents and I were in fits of laughter afterwards. Father declared, 'This is going to work. I just know it is!' and we ended up in a group hug and my words were, 'We'll show the buggers!'

Bill was a tremendous help. He took over the project because I was supposed to be resting. Bill saw to everything needed to get Adam started in business. He even got the Enterprise Allowance from the Job Centre for Adam. This would pay £40 per week for the first year. Flyers and leaflets were printed and posted through letter boxes and sent to organisations. The response was good.

In the first week Adam was open for business he had 32 cars to wash and valet. More than half of these cars came from police personnel – I wonder how that came about! The business went from strength to strength. Bill was always at the yard to help Adam move cars around after they had been washed, etc., but soon Adam became proficient at moving cars around and because the yard was private land it did not matter that he had not yet passed his driving test. There was so much for Adam to learn and everything had to be done and learned in a way suited to Adam's individuality, mainly through repetition. But, for the first time in his life, Adam was keen and interested. There was a problem with security!

The keys to any cars left by their owners needed to be secure. Adam had difficulty matching number plates with appropriate keys. So we had to stick a picture of an animal on the windscreen with a matching animal on the keys and the keys were locked in a cupboard in the shed. Likewise, Adam had a problem with time. So a car left in the morning and needed before lunch would have a picture of a cooked chicken placed on the windscreen, whilst a car left and not needed until teatime or after lunch had a picture of sandwiches placed on the windscreen.

Adam's business thrived. After the first two weeks he was able to buy a small second hand marquee so that he could work undercover in inclement weather.

Adam had problems understanding money. Initially, Bill was on hand to deal with payments but we worked out a system whereby the driver of the car would fill out the front of a specially printed envelope with their details and put the payment inside and Adam would lock the envelopes in a drawer in the shed. Similarly, we placed pictures on the windscreen for what was needed: a picture of a bucket for just a wash, a picture of a bucket and a tin of wax for wash and wax and a picture of a vacuum cleaner for a valet, etc.

Being involved with setting up the car wash business had taken my mind off my own problems somewhat. Constantly though, my future was on my mind. What was I going to do to earn money to pay our mortgage and to support my family?

I had been away from work for four months and I still received my full teaching salary but I knew this wouldn't go on forever. What was I going to do? Kathleen, my wife, and I discussed it frequently – we even talked about applying for disability benefits. But that wasn't the way I wanted to live. I needed to be independent, I needed to interact with other people, I needed a reason to get up in the morning. I continued to walk and talk to my dog, which was really therapeutic.

Out of the blue, I had a call from Cambridge University asking if I would lecture for them in the coming academic year. A week later a call came from Hertfordshire University. From these two calls and after hours of research, my business was formed – Focus disABILITY, offering training and consultation on all issues of disability. My first session at Cambridge was booked for a date in October and I knew I had to formally resign from my teaching job and get my G.P. to sign me as fit for work.

When I visited the G.P. and told him of my plan, he thought it a brilliant idea but said I wasn't ready for work as it would take time to wean me off the medication he had prescribed. He was really surprised when I told him I hadn't been taking the medication! Walking my dog and the wonder and beauty of nature took away the stress which had caused my burnout and I think I learned a valuable lesson from this experience. I learned that to take time to look at the beauty around us and really appreciate nature's power to heal and to rejuvenate! I also learned that classical and sacred music has therapeutic powers for me too!

I was able to reason with my G.P. through a long conversation and convinced him that I was recovered and ready to work again. I gained the medical certificate I needed to start earning my living again.

My head teacher was not very pleased when I handed in my resignation and to tell the truth, neither was I. So much had happened to me during my time at the school.

***

Two major events made a significant contribution to my life whilst at the school.

Not long before Christmas, a few years before I retired from teaching, I received a phone call informing me that a maiden aunt, who was eighty-five years of age, had been taken ill and was in hospital. I had been very close to this aunt in my younger years.

I travelled to Lancashire to see her. She refused to talk about herself. She had been deaf most of her life so communication had always been a little difficult. Although she wore hearing aids, she relied heavily on lip-reading but she was a forceful character, always outspoken and blunt! So I wasn't hurt when she commanded me:

'Alan, sit down, shut up and listen to me.'

I did as I was told.

'You have done well in life but there's one thing you've failed at! Do you know what that is?'

Oh dear, I thought was I in for a telling off. What had I failed to do? This aunt was notorious for speaking her mind to her extended family and all of my brothers and cousins had suffered her wrath at some time or another.

'Auntie, tell me what have I failed at?'

'You never passed your driving test. You gave up!'

'Auntie, you're going back thirty years or more!'

'I know, I know. But it's the only thing you've failed at and I want you to try again!'

In my late teens and early twenties I had taken driving lessons and after I'd failed about 8 or 9 driving tests I gave up.

'Auntie, I can't afford to drive again. I have a wife, a mortgage and teenage kids.'

'That's where you're wrong! Just you open that top drawer in my locker. There's a brown envelope in there with your name on it. Take it.'

I found the envelope and Auntie became excited and I could see she was watching my face.

'Well don't stand there dithering. Open it and look what's in it!'

I opened the envelope as requested and discovered a cheque made out to me for a substantial amount.

'What's this, Auntie? I can't take this!'

She placed her hand on mine and interrupted.

'Now shut up and listen. You are going to take that and you are going to take driving lessons and you're going to pass your driving test before I leave this earth!'

As she stopped to take a breath, I opened my mouth to speak but before I could say one word, Auntie held up her hand in a warning gesture!

'Now look here, Alan. I've asked you to shut up and listen to me. Don't argue. There's enough money there to pay for driving lessons and to buy a small car when you've passed your test. No arguments. Do it!'

All I could do was to thank her, for the stern and determined look was familiar to me. It conveyed domination – she meant it – I knew I had to obey!

It took four months for me to pass my driving test and buy a car! I learned to drive a car with automatic transmission which made it so much easier. These were not around in my early years.

One of my first journeys in my Renault 11 car was to Lancashire to visit my auntie, who was still in hospital. I parked my car outside the ward Auntie was on, hoping I could show her through a window what her money had bought.

As I entered the ward, there were three nurses trying to restrain my auntie who was making an awful noise! She had suffered a brain haemorrhage since my last visit and lost the ability to speak. As soon as I approached her bed, I could see what the problem was. I could see my car from the window adjacent to Auntie's bed and I assumed she had seen my arrival and had got over excited at the sight of me driving my car!

I really had to shout very loudly before the nurses released my auntie.

She threw herself at me and clung on to me and I knew it was her way of telling me how happy she was that I had passed my driving test.

I held her close, fighting my own emotions. It was so sad to see the deterioration in her and so difficult not to show how upset I was. Auntie had always been a rather robust woman of ample proportions but now her body was sparse of flesh and bent as opposed to the dignified erectness of her former years.

Suddenly, I had an idea! But I needed to speak with the sister of the ward before I could discuss my thinking with Auntie!

I found Sister in her office and introduced myself. I explained about my driving, my car and Auntie's part in this and then I asked, 'Sister, what's the possibility of me taking Auntie for a drive in my car?'

'Oh boy! I know she'd love that. But she would be so excited. I think we may have to scrape her off the ceiling when you tell her.'

Sister and I approached Auntie, who was sitting in a chair next to her bed. Auntie looked a little apprehensive as we walked towards her and she looked at me with a look which said, 'What have you done or what have you been up to?'

As we stood before her she inclined her head towards Sister who took her hand and stroked auntie's hair back from her face with a tenderness which was emotionally moving. Bending her body forward, her face to Auntie's eye level, she asked, 'Your nephew here would like to take you for a drive in his car. Would you like to go?'

I think the whole hospital heard the explosive whoop of wondrous joy which emitted from Auntie's throat. This was followed by the exaggerated nodding of the head.

Sister looked at me and exclaimed with a laugh, 'No doubt there. I should say she wants to go!'

'Auntie, try to calm down. Where would you like to go?'

I verbally listed a few places that I knew Auntie had frequently visited in her life. She had loved walking in the countryside. Almost every Saturday during my childhood she had walked with her friend and on occasions, after I had learned to walk, she had taken me with her too. I thought I knew her favourite spots but as I mentioned them one by one, she shook her head.

It was so frustrating and brought memories from the past when I was unable to speak. I knew what it was like and it was my turn to show patient acceptance as Auntie had done of me in the past.

I accompanied my next words by gently taking hold of Auntie's hand:

'I was thinking of driving up on a hill where you could see the countryside all around but you have somewhere else in mind?'

She nodded her head and pointed to pen and paper on her bedside.

She wrote Blackpool. Fish and chips!

This made Sister laugh, 'You want to go to Blackpool for fish and chips! That's at least a thirty mile drive. I think your nephew had a shorter trip in mind.'

'No, Sister, that's okay by me. If that's what she wants to do, we'll do it, providing it's alright by you!'

'We had better get you ready then, hadn't we?'

Auntie's face was beaming. She took up her pen again and wrote the word 'paper'.

'Yes Auntie – we'll take pen and paper with us.' And then I thought what I had said and the way I had said it may have sounded patronising. I was horrified. It was so easy to be patronising! Me patronising my beloved Auntie! I quickly forgave many people from my earlier years!

'I'm sorry Auntie. Did you mean can we take pen and paper?'

A shake of the head revealed that I had totally misunderstood.

She then wrote 'newspaper'.

'Newspaper!' I repeated whilst thinking deeply.

'Newspaper - You want to take a newspaper to read?'

Again, a shake of the head.

'I'm sorry. I'm not getting this, am I? I'm useless!' and then the light dawned, the penny dropped.

'Auntie, I have it now. You want to go to Blackpool and eat fish and chips out of newspaper on the promenade like we did years ago?'

The emphatic nod and the smiling face communicated that I had understood her correctly.

'We may have to sit in the car and eat our fish and chips rather than on a bench as we used to. Is that alright?'

She nodded her acceptance.

While one of the nursing staff got Auntie ready for the trip, I had time to think. Was Auntie trying to recreate or relive a trip we had often done together in my teenage years?

I was aware of a bit of a kerfuffle from behind the curtains which surrounded Auntie's bed as the nurse got her ready and when Auntie appeared, dressed in pale blue, her favourite colour, the nurse expressed surprise by exclaiming, 'Did you hear the fuss? All because she wanted to wear lipstick!'

Auntie was placed in a wheel chair and we began our journey through the ward to the car. Before we got to the door to go out from the ward, Auntie indicated that she wanted to turn around.

'Have you forgotten something?'

Her nod confirmed that she had. We travelled back to her bed and from her bedside drawer she removed her purse.

'You won't need money!'

A nod asserted that she would.

We got to the car and she got out of the wheelchair and, holding on to the car for support, she walked around it as though inspecting it.

'Do you like it? Do you approve, Auntie?'

A nod and the thumbs-up indicated that my choice of car met with her approval.

When we were both seated in the car, I explained what I intended to do, to make sure that Auntie and I had the same thing in mind.

'I'm going to park near the Manchester Hotel and get fish and chips from that shop near by. If it's still there! Is that what you want?'

I received a nod.

'Then when we've eaten our fish and chips, do you want to go Fleetwood way?'

A shake of the head!

'No. You want to go Lytham way?'

A nod of the head!

As we were driving along, she touched the wedding ring on my finger and, without taking my eyes off the road, I explained that Kathleen was well. I also talked about my children.

I was concerned that she couldn't hear me over the noise of the car engine but her hearing aids seemed to be working really well!

At one point in the journey I thought she became fidgety, but when I looked she was merely turning this way and that, looking around the car.

'You really like the car. It's comfortable, isn't it?'

59

I could see big tears rolling down her cheeks so I pulled over and parked by the kerb.

'What's up, Auntie?'

She extended her forearms from her elbows, with palms upward and, using shoulder movements and eye movements, conveyed her thoughts.

'You're just happy to see me driving; is that it?'

A nod, a beaming smile and a slap on my thigh told me I was right.

We resumed our journey and Auntie pointed out familiar spots and I verbalised for her.

We arrived in Blackpool and I parked the car and eventually started to move from my seat to go and get the fish and chips. My progress was stopped by Auntie taking quite a heavy grip on my arm and I resumed my position in the driver's seat.

'Now what's up? If you're going to ask if you can drive the car back, the answer's no!'

This jibe was met by shining eyes, a smile and rather a hefty punch on my upper left arm.

I saw her fiddling in her purse. Obviously she wanted to pay for the fish and chips!

'Auntie, hold on. How much have you in your purse?'

She looked at me indignantly! It was a 'What's it got to do with you?' look.

'You know we've forgotten something, don't you?'

A frown and hand movements conveyed that she didn't understand.

'We used to have fish and chips and then go to Pablo's!'

This was met by a beaming smile which involved her eyes and I took it to mean a visit to Pablo's was accepted. (Pablo's was a famous ice-cream parlour in Blackpool and we used to go there each time we visited the town.)

Auntie demanded that she pay for the fish and chips and we ate them while parked, overlooking the sea. I was amazed at how much she ate and she insisted I ate what she had left. All through her life she had lived by the motto 'waste not, want not' and I supposed that was in her mind as she bade me eat her leftover fish and chips!

Next stop was Pablo's and I thoroughly enjoyed watching her tuck into a large multi-flavoured ice-cream.

As I pushed her in her wheelchair from Pablo's, she indicated that she wanted to go left from the shop. The car was to the right! I could not think where she wanted to go. I pushed her according to her directions and she took me to a shop where they made Blackpool rock on the premises. I was surprised she had remembered it. I had forgotten it.

She purchased quite a lot of rock and I wondered who it was for, but I didn't question. She was obviously enjoying herself and I didn't want to spoil her pleasure.

We then travelled along the coast road to Lytham and St Annes and I was told in no uncertain terms where to park. We sat in silence overlooking the sea and Auntie looked so relaxed and so contented. I reclined my seat, much to Auntie's wonder, and reclined her seat for her and we both fell asleep.

We did not get back to the hospital until 7:30 in the evening and I apologised to Sister but she said it didn't matter and that it was good to see Auntie looking so happy.

All the rock she bought – I should have guessed. As I left, Auntie was sat in the chair by the side of her bed, handing out sticks of Blackpool rock to all the nurses.

That was the last time I saw Auntie alive but the memories of the circumstances of my learning to drive and of the trip to Blackpool are rather poignant to me.

Was it coincidence that I learned to drive at that time? I could never even have contemplated starting my business had Auntie not have given me the means of learning to drive. I'm also forcibly reminded that I am as I am through the support and the patience of not only my immediate family but my extended family as well.

I have enjoyed driving! Not only did it become necessary in earning my living, it also allowed me to take advantage of many opportunities. Because I had a car and I was able to drive, I was able to expand opportunities for many of the pupils I taught in school. I could ferry them around to work placements or help them to attend course in colleges. Previously these placements had been restricted to a walking distance from school.

***

I was really shocked when I was approached by a theatre group who wanted to turn my published autobiography into a play for education! (My first autobiography, *So Clean in My Mind*, was published in October, 1982.)

After permission had been given I was involved as a coach/consultant and it was exciting to see my life story unfold on the stage.

Because I was able to drive, I could attend many performances around the country and I was introduced to the audience at the end of each performance I attended. The purpose of the production and my appearance was to raise awareness and I enjoyed being a part of this. I could never have been as involved as I was had I not have been able to drive. I learned many things about myself during this time as I answered questions, some of them personal, from people in the audience. Some of these questions caused me to do some soul searching and I developed and became a better person through the experience.

Coincidentally, the date of the first performance of the play was the day I passed my driving test.

These memories and experiences are linked to my period of employment at the last school I taught at. Having to retire and giving in my notice of termination were very traumatic for many reasons!

***

Having secured that final medical certificate which I needed to resume employment, I visited the Job Centre to ask for advice on and apply for Enterprise Allowance. There had been a recession in the early 1980s and so many people had lost their jobs and were claiming unemployment benefit. Margaret Thatcher's government introduced the Enterprise Allowance Scheme, which paid £40 per week, to encourage people who were unemployed to become self-employed. I wasn't sure whether this scheme applied to me as I had lost my job through ill health rather than through the recession. I was interviewed by a woman who was so patronising and negative. The attitude of this woman annoyed me. She constantly referred to my disability, she suggested I should apply for disability benefits and suggested that with my limitations I should not be even thinking of working. I was proud of my history of employment but this awful woman did not mention my former employment experience or my qualifications. Her conversation led me to believe she saw my disability and ignored my ability. Her comments really angered me. But it was the last straw when she said:

'Well you appear intelligent and I can tell you've really thought about your business plan. But it can't work! How can you trade as a trainer? You have awful speech – you have a speech impediment!'

Making the necessary effort, I raised my voice and after an audible intake of breath and expressing sarcastic surprise, I angrily replied.

'I have a speech impediment! I have a speech impediment! I have lived 50 years and now you tell me I have a speech impediment. I never knew I had a speech impediment. I am devastated! I've been teaching most of my life and now you tell me I have a speech impediment. Wow. I really don't know what to say. I've been sitting here talking to you for forty minutes; never once have you asked me to repeat myself and I've answered all your questions and you have answered mine. I thought you understood what I was saying because you responded to everything I said but now you tell me, at my age and after all my experience of employment, I have awful speech and a speech impediment! What a revelation!'

Obviously the woman wasn't pleased with my sarcasm and turned down my application for Enterprise Allowance! But as I was leaving the Job Centre I was invited to join another woman in a cubicle adjacent to the one I'd been interviewed in.

'Mr Counsell, come and talk to me.'

I entered her cubicle and sat opposite her at her desk.

'Mr Counsell, this is not very professional of me but I heard much of your interview in there,' she said, indicating the next cubicle. 'I want to help you. Can you leave me your application, your business plan and your business brochure and can you come back and see me in two days time? Make it late afternoon. I need time to speak to a few people.' She handed me her business card.

I returned to the Job Centre as requested and was asked to wait in reception. I waited for quite some time before I was invited into an office, not a cubicle this time but an enclosed office. I was introduced to a man sat behind a desk who was immaculate in appearance and who exuded an air of authority. Immediately my mental processes went into defensive mode and I was ready to pounce at the first negative comment he should make.

'Mr Counsell. Come in, sit down and relax. May I call you Alan? My name is John and I am from the local office of The Training and Enterprise Council.'

The Training and Enterprise Councils were set up in the late 1980s by the Thatcher government to help England and Wales recover from recession. Part of the remit of Training and Enterprise Councils was to promote business enterprise. They had public funding and reported to central government.

John's first comment to me put me at ease and made me relax.

'Alan, I really want you to forget your visit to this office a few days ago. We are not going to discuss it. I have to tell you, you have been awarded the Enterprise Allowance. I just need to know what date you would like that to begin and what bank account you would like it to be paid into?'

I was rather speechless and all I could do was to thank him.

We decided on a date. October 8th 1990. During that week I had a day's lecturing booked for Cambridge University. They became my first client and October 8th 1990 is the date I became officially self-employed.

John's second comment surprised me too.

'We have assigned you a business councillor from the local Chamber of Commerce and I need to set up a time when you can meet with him.'

We discussed a time and John used the telephone to arrange for me to meet with my business councillor.

Again, I could only thank John! I was speechless! But there was more!

'Alan, we have enrolled you on a training course for Business Start Ups and the Chamber of Commerce, who run the course, will send you details and arrange everything with you.'

At this stage in my meeting with John I was feeling a bit of an idiot because all I could say was thank you and I was aware that I was repeating myself but I didn't know what else to say.

But then came the biggest surprise of all!

'Now, Alan, You know you're not unknown locally. Your fame has gone before you. All the community work you did involving your students when you were teaching is well-known. So based on your reputation, I can commission you to do one day's training a month for the next twelve months. Obviously we need to discuss the content of that training but based on your C.V. and your business brochure we want you to train for us. Now, how much are you going to charge me for a day's training?'

I really wasn't prepared. I had come to this meeting expecting it to be solely about the Enterprise Allowance Scheme. So I was a bit flummoxed by the additional business. However, I do have the ability to think on the hoof so I quickly recovered myself, assumed a business-like manner and asked a few questions which I thought made me appear intelligent and aware.

'John, I need to know how long a training day you want? I need to know how many people will attend the training day? I also need to know where the training venue will be before I can give you a costing.'

He had to think but eventually he answered all my questions and I was able to give him some options. I had a basic price for a certain number of people on the course if the number exceeded that which I had quoted, then the cost was more. Likewise if I had to produce handouts for the people attending the course, then I would levy an additional charge. There was an option for each of my clients to produce their own handouts from my master copies; this was a cheaper option. If I had to travel over 15 miles from my home to a training venue then I also charged travel costs.

I think the way I reacted to John's offer of a commission was impressive. I was impressed by myself. And maybe I appeared organised and prepared. I felt good.

John and I agreed numbers, cost and venues and even booked dates for the first three training days.

I left the Job Centre and sat in my car, tingling with excitement. I couldn't wait to tell Kathleen all that had happened at my meeting with John. I found it difficult to believe that all my plans, which Kathleen had helped me to formulate, were coming to fruition. I felt I was in a dream. It was as though there had been divine intervention and I just knew my new venture was going to be a success. I was aware that I could be too excited and over-optimistic while Kathleen was always level-headed and down to earth; she always reasoned with me and made me see reality. But on this occasion, as I explained all about my day on her return from work, she shared all my feelings and, holding me in her arms, she really boosted my already soaring confidence by saying:

'I believe in you. You succeed in everything you do. You are great and I feel so lucky to have you. I love you so much!' and, releasing me from her hold, she added, 'Your business plan will work and I know you are going to keep me in the manner and custom I've yet to grow accustomed to!'

And so it was! My business was launched!

Ironically, the dog that had come into my life at the beginning of my illness, without me planning for it or even wanting it, but had played a major part in my recovery from professional burnout, had to be put down at this time because he became very ill. My farewell was very emotional. It seemed that Sooty the poodle had come into my life when I needed a silent companion with whom I could verbalise my thoughts to, while employing my emotional powers to reason my way through a grim time in my life. Now I was better and ready to move on, it seemed Sooty had served his purpose and moved on too!

As a delegate on the fourth training course I did for the local Training and Enterprise Council, I had the first woman I saw at the Job Centre, the one who turned down my application for Enterprise Allowance. It took a great deal of willpower on my part for me not to pick on her. As a trainer, I was aware of the power I had. But I ignored my natural feelings for revenge and allowed her to be just another delegate, but being human, I really couldn't let the opportunity go without a jibe! At the end of the day I made a public statement to the assembled group!

'Ladies and gentlemen, thank you for coming today. I've really enjoyed working with you and I want to share something personal and maybe emotional with you. As a child, I could not speak and I struggled and worked so hard to acquire speech. I was well into my teens before people really understood my speech. What a thrill it is to stand before you this day and know you have all understood what I have said to you, for you have all responded to me without ever having asked me to repeat myself. I know you've had to listen carefully and maybe concentrate a little more than you normally would and I thank you for your attention. I feel a remarkable sense of achievement.'

Many people came forward and the consensus of opinion was that my speech was easy to understand and I hoped 'my friend' heard these comments.

Right from the start my business was a success and I was busy. At the time I started my business there were 19 training and enterprise councils established in England and Wales and the majority commissioned me to train for them. As my reputation grew, I got more and more work. I travelled extensively, facilitating training courses or consulting or counselling individuals. I had so much work that during my second year of trading, Kathleen gave up her job as a classroom assistant at a local school and joined me in the business.

It was as though someone somewhere was really looking after us. We were concerned about leaving our fourteen-year-old daughter home alone whilst we were away working – many days on residential courses and often in hotels. The vet who had attended Sooty visited to tell us that a local kennel had asked him to put one of their dogs down because she had become too old to breed! The vet was not happy and asked if we would consider taking this dog into our home as a pet. So Gemma, the wired haired fox terrier, came to live with us. After the first few days she showed herself to be an excellent guard dog and proved to be a protector for our daughter when we weren't at home.

Gemma was a wonderful solution to our worries!

Whilst out shopping in the City Centre on one of my infrequent days off, my wife and I met a woman who was vaguely familiar to me. It was a face from my past and my memory struggled to recognise who she was and where I knew her from. As we exchanged pleasantries, I fought to recollect who she was. She obviously knew me but could I bring her to mind? Rather than ask who she was, I let her speak, hoping she would give some clue. She mentioned the school I used to work at and she mentioned the hospital and suddenly the penny dropped. She was the paediatrician from the hospital who had attended the children at the school and we had met fleetingly in the past as our paths crossed in our professional duties.

I did not know her very well. I don't recall ever having had a conversation with her before. But here she was talking to me as though we were good friends. She knew I'd left teaching and she knew I was working for myself. She asked if I would like to do some casual work for her at the hospital. We set up a meeting for a few days hence. And so it came to be that I was appointed as a counsellor to the paediatric department at the local hospital. My remit was very specific! I worked with mothers who had given birth to a child with disability. I also worked with the families of the child too! This was a new venture for the hospital. Previously the midwives and nurses had been involved and they did a really good job.

I was a little apprehensive because my counselling qualification was from 1963 and this was 1992. I was also out of practice as a counsellor and did not carry any insurance.

But my friendly paediatrician was adamant that I was the man she wanted. I accepted the assignment, provided I could get insurance and provided I had support! The fee offered was very small too but I had previously said when setting up my business that I would rather work for pennies than sit at home not earning anything and I had learned from experience that the more people I worked with, the more my reputation grew and one never knew who was going to book the next course!

It was interesting to meet new parents. I made a point to 'coo' over the disabled baby and I was sincere in enjoying my contact with each new life. I was so surprised at the issues the mums and dads needed to talk about! Maybe my past experience hadn't prepared for these counselling sessions but I very quickly learned. The majority of parents were scared. Somehow being told that their child had disability had taken away the joy of the birth of a new life and had brought fear. Some disabilities had been diagnosed even before birth through scans and other tests. Expectant mothers of these foetuses would receive counselling, usually towards abortion, and I did so admire those who decided to keep their child even though they knew the child would be born with a disability. Personally I am totally against abortion, particularly if it's because something has been detected in the unborn child which might cause a disability. It leads me to think, 'should I have been born?' I believe I have contributed to society and many of my friends with congenital disabilities have made valuable contributions. But there are those who would advise abortion had our disabilities been detected before birth.

I do know that a new mother might experience fear because motherhood is a new experience but the parents I met (sometimes experienced parents) would express fear around the disability aspect of caring and nurturing their child. It was interesting to learn that parents have all kinds of expectation for and of the child even before the child is born. Many a mother told me of her vision and expectation of her daughter as a bride and because her daughter had been born with disability that expectation had been dashed. This always surprised me and my mental question was always, 'Why can't a disabled woman wear a beautiful bridal gown?' I never asked that question but I did ask other questions which evoked thought from the parents. Ultimately, I wanted these parents to see their disabled children as individuals and celebrate the uniqueness of their children but always the parents would raise questions about how their child might be accepted and treated by the extended family and by society in general. The babies I saw would be around a month old by the time I saw their parents. Fathers were usually concerned about the impact a disabled child might have on their image and on what others might think of them because of their child, whilst most grandparents were keen to tell me that there was nothing 'like that' on their side of the family!

Many parents would question me about my own disability and my own childhood but I was reluctant to tell much about myself for I did not want to raise false hopes, nor did I want to detract from the real issues which were that my clients were now the parents of a baby who had been diagnosed with disability.

The majority of parents would tell me of the confidence they had in me because I knew all about it as a result of my own disability. Many said they would be happy if their child grew up to be like me and that caused me concern. Each child was unique with their own individual potential and I was always concerned that the parents might see me as a role model and develop unrealistic ambitions!

I wasn't sure my counselling sessions did any good. Most parents would book more sessions with me and my supervisor gave positive feedback but I could not see or judge the results of my work. I had lots of comments from parents about health visitors and social workers, about how parents felt they were constantly watched, how parents' privacy was often invaded and the many issues around this.

My role was very different to that of health visitor or a social worker. It seemed that all the services offered to parents at that time were child-oriented. I was parent-oriented. I was there to get families, especially parents, talking together about their thoughts and feelings. My aims were decided by each family and often by each individual in that family. I was amazed at the issues that came up in our sessions and I came to know the value of my services as there were not many other agencies offering a similar service. With many of my parents, I knew that the opportunity they had to talk about issues which arose from my questions could and would prevent a future divorce!

Initially I would explain that I was there for them. I wasn't there to give advice on the child. I would always begin by asking, 'Is there anything you want to talk about?' Usually I got little response to this but just a simple question, 'How do you feel about giving birth to a disabled child?' and my insistence on an answer could produce some soul-searching and usually opened up a dialogue. I heard many husbands and wives say to each other, 'I didn't know you felt like that!' There followed a very meaningful discussion that ignored me. I would only intervene if there was misunderstanding or confrontation. I would always try to initiate a discussion on need, for, from experience, I had found that many husbands and wives were oblivious to the needs of the other in dealing with their thoughts, feelings and indeed trauma in being the new parents of a disabled child.

With so many parents commenting on the services of health visitors and social workers, I asked the hospital authority if an evening's course could be arranged for health visitors, social workers and parents, so we might discuss the issues and concerns in a forum. The powers that be accepted the idea but on the evening of the course eight parents turned up, but just one health visitor. I thought that was rather telling! I was more than willing to facilitate such a course during the day but apparently health visitors and social workers could not be released from work for such a course!

People talk, word gets around, reputations and comparisons are made and through one of my mothers who came to me for counselling I was introduced to a young woman named June who lived locally. It was suggested that I could help this young woman through my counselling skills. I didn't like this kind of referral as I was always reluctant to ask for a fee, I never knew how much time it might involve and was concerned that I might be so busy with my training assignments that I may not have the time to do a good job. But the words of my mother were ever with me:

'If you can help others and forget yourself you'll gain from the experience'. And really I had so much in my life and I wanted and needed to give something back.

June was nineteen years of age and had been involved in a road traffic accident two years earlier. She was a beauty. She had the most gorgeous of blue eyes and a turned-up nose. Her long blonde hair had a natural curl and it cascaded around her shoulders. She didn't wear makeup and although her complexion was relatively good I thought it lacked a little care. As with all counselling, the aim is to get the client to talk about their personal issues and help them to find solutions from within themselves. I chatted to June at the start of our first appointment about things in general to allow June to get to know me and tune in to my speech.

I then asked, 'Tell me, how do you go from being one person one minute – the person you've been for seventeen years – to being a different person because you've been hit by a car?'

She looked at me with eyes wide open, appeared stunned and after a little silence she haltingly exclaimed.

'That's it! That's what I want to talk about. You understand, don't you? Nobody else has asked me that and that's what I want to talk about!'

Somehow the hour-long session stretched into two as the floodgates opened and June talked and talked and talked.

Amazingly, June came to her third session wearing light makeup and looking absolutely stunning! I did comment on her appearance and got her to talk about fashion and jewellery and things my own teenage daughters talked about.

We had previously talked about 'scriptwriting' and expectation. I believe we all have a mental script for life and the basis for that script might be formed in our childhood. We plan out our life in our minds as we grow and we adjust our plan and rewrite our script as we experience life. We also have an identity. June's identity had always been of a non-disabled person and most of her expectations and experience were around this identity. In her formative years she had developed a very negative attitude towards 'disability' and towards 'disabled people'. Now, she was one! Because of her negative thinking around disability before being hit by the car, she was confused about who she was and what she was.

As we went through our weekly sessions it became obvious that she was taking on board the many and complex issues involved in changing one's identity. Her statement, 'I might have changed but I've still got a life to live!' signalled to me that maybe my job was done and June no longer needed me.

But June asked if I thought she could ever work and how she should go about finding a job. I simply directed her to the local Job Centre and a disablement resettlement officer.

June and I had several counselling sessions after she had attended the Job Centre; ultimately June decided she didn't need counselling anymore and we parted company.

It was during one of the balmy, Indian summer evenings which we sometimes experience in our English autumn that the doorbell rang and there stood Adam and his mum, both grinning like Cheshire cats. I hadn't seen Adam very much during the past six months or so because I'd been very busy with my own business but I knew he was doing exceedingly well in every way. Mother and son stood at my door and their body language and their general aura conveyed great excitement.

'What's up, said I, 'Are you coming in?'

And as they entered my home I asked, 'Where's dad?'

They both started to giggle and couldn't answer my question. I'm afraid I'm prone to giggling myself. Giggling is contagious, a bit like yawning – but I controlled myself and tried to be stern.

'What's going on?' I asked, 'And where's dad? Did you walk here?'

It took mum a little while to compose herself and with a mischievous look on her face and whilst wiping tears from her cheeks she offered:

'No, we didn't walk here and we've left him at home!' and after she tapped Adam on his arm and indicated by head movements that he should speak, Adam exclaimed in great excitement:

'I've passed my driving test today and I had to come and tell you!'

Not only am I prone to giggles, I am also a very emotional person as well. So, with tears flowing down my cheeks, I gathered them both to my chest and added to the electrifying atmosphere they had brought into my home. I think I had every right to feel joyful and to express that joy by shedding tears - I did have a small part to play in this man's success!

We did eventually calm down but mother didn't help by saying:

'I can't believe it, my Adam...'

I was led to reflect that many months ago when I first met Adam, no one could have anticipated the progress, the development and the remarkable achievements of this young man. The comparison between then and now was extraordinarily noticeable. He had come from being an introverted couch potato with little interest in life, a very selfish and negative being to someone with vitality and zest, with an obvious personality and character. He carried himself very erect and he now had a body rippling with muscle. His hair was cut in a modern way, still curly but flopping over his forehead, bringing a look of innocence and charm to his smiling and twinkling eyes. He exuded confidence! It was a joy to see him! He still walked with a limp and still had a clumsy hand but these were less obvious because of his improved attitude. There was also an obvious affection and a much closer relationship between mother and son and that was good to see too.

We sat talking for a while and I was so impressed by Adam. His conversation was more mature and relevant. He spoke very enthusiastically about his business and his future plans, one of which was to get someone to work with him because he was so busy and needed someone to help with the administration side of things. I was too busy with my own work to be of much help but I did phone Bill and asked him to help by visiting the Job Centre and the local Chamber of Commerce to gather information about employing people.

I then had an idea!

I hadn't seen June for a few weeks and I knew the last time I saw her she was visiting the Job Centre to look for work. Was it possible that June could be Adam's girl Friday? I contacted June and discovered she hadn't got a job but was attending a college course, studying business studies in the evening. I introduced June to Bill and Adam and the four of us talked and introduced the needs of the business. At the conclusion of our meeting and after a brief and whispered conversation with Adam, Bill asked June if she would accept a job at the car wash if one was offered to her. Her whole body language replied rather positively. I'm sure Adam wasn't aware of his reaction to June but it led me to think: was Adam a ladies' man?

And so it came to be that June found employment with Adam. I couldn't visit the car wash very often but Bill kept me informed of how things were going. It didn't take but a month for Bill to contact me and tell me he felt redundant as June had reorganised the admin and had everything under control.

It was good to hear.

One has to remember that Adam had learning difficulty with a very limited experience of life, while June's injuries had caused her to be very shy and insular and she forced herself to do things and integrate with the general public. Her injuries had caused her to have epilepsy and a drooping eyelid and although this was not pronounced to others, it was a major impairment to June, a young woman. I think too that because June had a very well groomed and sophisticated mother and two sisters, one older, one younger, who were both 'drop dead' gorgeous, who wore the latest fashion, including high heeled shoes which June couldn't wear because of a spinal injury, caused June to compare herself to her family and to have a very unrealistic and negative mental image of herself.

So the car wash became the prime interest in life for both her and Adam. Adam was taught how to care for June and what to do should June have an epileptic episode whilst at work. Bill was very often at the car wash and Adam's family were quite near too.

So it was three months into this partnership between Adam and June that he came to see me in my home. He did complain that I was never home and that he had been four times before. I told him he should telephone before he visited then he would know when I was home.

To which he replied, 'I can't use the telephone!'

I was a little surprised and made a mental note to look into this at a later date. I guessed Adam had come for a purpose and I didn't want to distract him. I was so shocked when Adam asked if he could speak with me in private! Previously he hadn't a concept of 'private' or 'public' so I took him into the dining room and closed all the doors. But I was further surprised when my oldest daughter teased Adam by saying:

'I'm going to listen through the door.'

To which he replied very quickly, no thinking time:

'You were always a nosey bugger and it's a glass door so I'll stop talking if I see you.'

It takes intelligence and awareness to make that kind of comment and observation. The Adam I knew didn't have these traits. He was indeed developing!

'What do you want to see me about?' I asked.

'It's about June.'

'What about June?'

73

'She's great!' Thereby followed a silence

'Adam, I know June is great. But what do you want to talk about?'

'It's about June.'

'Right Adam, it's about June. Do you have a problem with June?'

'No!' Silence again.

'Adam, I'm not a mind reader. Has June got a problem you want to talk about?'

'What's a mind reader?'

'Tell me about June. Tell me why you came to see me?'

'Do you think I'll ever get married? My brother's getting married but he says nobody will have me. So when mum and dad die I'll have to go and live with him and his wife. I don't want mum and dad to die and I don't want to live with my brother!'

'Wow, Adam, that's a bit cruel of your brother but he was being very kind. He is saying he really cares about you and he wants to look after you. That's nice, isn't it?'

'But I don't need looking after. Not by him anyway. And I don't want mum and dad to die.'

'Adam. Tell me, are your mum and dad young or old?'

'My mum and dad are young aren't they? My grandma's old!'

'Do young people die, Adam?'

'No. Grandpa died and he was very old.'

'Right, Adam! So maybe your mum and dad won't die until they're old like grandpa was.'

'Oh, that's good.'

'Adam, Grandpa died and he was old. Grandma is old. Who looks after grandma?'

'Grandma lives with my auntie and uncle because they look after her. My mum says it's a good job grandma lives there because she couldn't look after herself.'

'And your brother is saying a long time from now, if you need someone to look after you, he and his new wife will do it. That's nice to know, isn't it?'

'But I don't need looking after!'

'That's good! But if you did, your brother's offered!'

I could see Adam was thinking about what I had said and I gave him time to assimilate.

Eventually, I broke the silence.

'Are you okay, Adam? Do you want to talk some more or do you understand?'

'I feel better about my brother – in a way – but he was nasty because he said no one would have me!'

'Can we deal with that later, Adam, because I'm not happy! This is hard for me. I think you are thinking people only die when they're older and I know a few people who have died when they were younger.'

'My dog died and he was only three and my dad said these things happen and we deal with them when they happen. So if my mum and dad die before they are old, we will have to deal with it and my brother will be there to help me.'

I am happy with Adam's reasoning and somewhat relieved because the coward within me didn't want to answer the awkward questions of 'What happens when you die?' or 'Why do people die?' or 'Where do people go when they die?' But I was not prepared for Adam's next questions.

'Alan, you're married. Do you think I can get married? That's why I want to talk to you!'

'Is that why you wanted to talk about June?'

I could see tears in his eyes and I felt his discomfort and embarrassment.

'Right, we are going to take this slowly. Tell me why you are upset. It's alright to cry. You've seen me cry and I want you to tell me everything, then we can sort it out for you. Now what's making you cry?'

'Because my dad says I'm a nuisance.'

'Why are you a nuisance to your dad?'

'No, I'm not a nuisance to my dad. I'm a nuisance to June!'

I had to think for a minute. I knew it was sometimes difficult for Adam to explain his thoughts and feelings and it was difficult for me to understand and follow his conversation. After a brief silence, I said:

'Adam, I'm going to sit here and listen to you. I want you to talk and talk and talk and I'll talk when you've finished!'

So Adam talked and it soon became obvious what the issues were!

Apparently, Adam collected June in his car every morning for work and took her home at the end of the day. Often he would stay and have a meal with June's family and sometimes June would have an evening meal with Adam's family. Dad thought Adam was spending too much time with June – possibly making a nuisance of himself!

'Well, Adam!' I said in a pause in Adam's talking. 'What can we do about this?'

'I don't know. Dad says I've to give June space. I spend too much time with her!'

'Okay. Tell me, what do you do when you've finished work?'

'Monday, Wednesday and Friday, I go to the gym and then I go home and watch telly.'

'Is that all you do?'

There was a silence and I could see Adam thinking.

'No, but if I tell you, you won't have a go at me like my parents do, will you? I think I'm sensible and I do what Bill says.'

'Adam, just talk to me. I'm not going to have a go. Just tell me.'

'Well, after gym on Friday I go to the bar and have a game of darts and a drink with Dave (Dave being my friend, the manager of the leisure centre where the gym is) and my dad and mum don't like it because they say I should not drink and sometimes I don't get home until very late because we get hungry and we get fish and chips or a McDonald's and mum goes bananas because I'm late home and mum won't go to bed until I get home. And the other thing is that my dad came to get me last Friday at the bar and June was there. Dad was really angry that June was there and I don't know why he shouted at me.'

There was a silence. I just waited. Adam continued.

'I didn't ask June to come. She turns up.' Another silence, more tears.

'I don't want to get rid of June. I don't want a man working at the garage. I want June. She makes me laugh and I make her laugh and we both enjoy working together. I like being with June I want to be with her all the time!'

This was followed by a silence and a few more tears and I thought there might be more for Adam to say, so I encouraged Adam to go on talking by asking:

'Adam, why should you get rid of June?'

He explained that dad thought he should have a man working at the car wash and not June, and this was evidently distressing to Adam.

I needed more information, so I asked Adam to talk more and to tell me where Bill came into all this. Because he had said previously, 'I do what Bill says!'

'Bill says I should never take my car with me if I'm going to have a drink and I don't. I leave my car at home on Fridays when I go to the gym. Dave thinks I'm silly because I never drink more than two lemonade shandies. Dave says I'll be alright to drive on that but I do what Bill says.'

'Why does your dad want you to get rid of June?'

'Because I like June and she likes me and I told my dad I want to marry her and dad says that could never be and it would be better if I got rid of June because I'm going to get very hurt. But I say if my brother can get married, why can't I?'

'Adam, I'm on your side but I think we need to talk about this! What do you think June's mum and dad would say if you told them you wanted to marry their daughter?'

'June's mum and dad like me! I know they do! They keep on telling me that I'm good for June. Her mum says June hasn't had one fit since she's worked at the car wash and she's really happy when she comes home from work. I think her sisters like me as well. I think they'd like me to marry her. I'm not daft. I know I need to save up for a house but I'm already doing that. That's another thing with my parents too, Alan; when I was younger they got benefits for me and they still get them and I think they get enough, I don't want to pay them every week. I want to save my money. I'm not telling June I want to marry her yet. I want to wait. Dave and my mates at the gym think we're too young and we need to have a good time before I get married. I know what I'm doing. June can't have babies because of the car crash. Something happened to her and she can't have babies. I haven't told my dad that because that's private. isn't it? When I've sorted myself out I'm going to take June out to a meal and to concerts and to the pictures, I'm not ready yet but I soon will be. Can June drink wine because of her epilepsy? I'm not taking my car when June and I go out for a meal in case we have wine. Dave said if I ask June out for a meal, he'd take us in his car and my other mates at the gym have dared me to ask June out. They say if I ask her, they will pay for a meal but if I don't I have to take them out for a meal.'

'Wow, Adam, I'm really impressed. Tell me what you mean when you say, "when I've sorted myself out and that you're not ready yet"?'

77

Adam looks at the floor in embarrassment. I have to encourage.

'Come on, Adam. Tell me, I'm your friend?'

'It's my gammy hand. I can't cut food. I can't use a knife and I don't know what to do. I could ask the waiter to cut my food for me or I could ask June but I don't want to and that's what I mean. I'm shy because of my hand.'

'Hey Adam, I have a hand too. Have you seen me cut up my food? Then maybe you could copy me! Don't you ever be ashamed of any thing about you. Be proud of yourself. You're doing well! What do you want to do now? Do you want to talk some more or learn how to use a knife?'

Adam decided he wanted to learn how to use a knife. It was so simple. Adam just held his knife as I held mine and within seconds he was able to cut through a thick crust of bread.

'Alan, that's magic. I'll have to practice but I'm excited! Your hand is worse than mine because you have a peg on the steering wheel of your car and I don't and if you can cut your food up, I can.'

The phone rang and it was Adam's mum. I heard Adam's response. 'Mum, I'm with Alan. It's 9 o'clock, I'll be ages yet. I'm nearly 20. I bet Geoff isn't in and he is not 18 yet. Have you rung him? ... Mum, I'm always up for work. I'll be home when I've finished here. Bye!'

We talked some more and I was more than assured that Adam knew what he was doing. We worked out a strategy for him to follow: it involved him believing in himself so that he is not upset when unkind things are said to him; it involved taking his dad with him of a Friday evening for a drink because I knew it would do dad good to see Adam with his mates in the bar at the gym; it involved talking to mum and dad about money and benefits and it involved asking Bill to look at bank accounts to make sure they were safe. I had no idea who the signatures are for cheques and withdrawals, etc. We also talked about the problems of taking June out to a meal. Adam can't read! Who's going to read the menu and the wine list to him?

Two days later I received a phone call from Adam's dad to tell me that Adam had been laying down the law about who decides what friends he has and the money he was giving mum each week and the time he came home at night. Adam's dad was surprised at the way Adam explained things and he felt Adam knew his own mind and had put over his points in a way that mum and dad couldn't argue! His dad asked if learning difficulty was curable and of course it isn't but when the authorities label people, they don't take personality and character into account and they don't really know how people react to life's experiences. When Adam was diagnosed, like most children with congenital disabilities, the diagnosis is based on the outcome of general tests which measure against a set of norms. The tests never take into account individuality, or personality, background or even character! Adam still had learning difficulty but he had so much ability which compensated for his problems.

It wasn't long before Adam rang me! Adam rang me! I thought he couldn't use the phone.

'Alan, I did it!'

'Adam, what did you do?'

'I took June out for a meal last night and it was good. Every thing went well. June can't drink because of her medication so the wine was no problem and I cut up my own meat and I paid from my wallet and told the man to keep the change!'

'Well, I'm really impressed. Sounds like you did well.'

'Course I did well. I'm sorry you weren't home on Friday. I tried to get you on the telephone then but you were out. So Dave took me out!'

'Just explain that to me again please. I'm not understanding you. You said you rang me last Friday. How? You told me you couldn't use the phone!'

'Oh, I can't. I get someone else to dial the number and I speak when they answer!'

'So you got someone to dial my number and I was not in. So Dave took you out. Explain it please.'

'Well, Dave dialled your number for me. I wanted to go out for a meal, to practice before I took June out. But you weren't in. So Dave took me instead. Dave said he knew your favourite place and he took me there. It was really good because when I took June I didn't need the menu; I just had what I had on Friday and it looked like I could read. Dave came to the car wash and put money in two wallets. If June had wine, I had to pay from a big wallet and get the change back but if June had the set meal like I had with no wine, I took the money from the little wallet and told the waiter to keep the change. And June had the same meal I had and it was easy peasy.'

'Well, I'm really happy for you... No I'm not, you little monkey. You took my mate Dave to my favourite restaurant – I'm jealous!'

Through giggles, I heard, 'I know Dave said you would be and I love making you jealous!'

I couldn't believe this young man. He understood and returned with humour!

'I can't wait till Friday.'

'Why, Adam, Are you taking June out again?'

'No, Alan, I'm not taking June out. I've got the receipt for the meal in my pocket and I'm going to give it to my mates. They said they would pay if I took June out for a meal. I'm not daft. They will have to pay up. I'll show the buggers!'

Well. That really made me laugh but I wasn't prepared for the next comment.

'You know, Alan, Dave might be your mate but he better keep his mouth shut on Friday. Can you tell me any stories about Dave that will shut him up?'

'Adam, you will have to explain a little more. What will Dave have to keep his mouth shut about?'

'Well we weren't in the restaurant or the car park when Dave came for us and when we got to the car he wanted to know where we'd been and June blushed and I told her not to and I just said we'd been for a walk in the garden and Dave said it was dark so why had we been in the garden and June blushed again. I told Dave to mind his own business but he teased us all the way home. How do I shut him up?'

I could not answer for laughing but I finally said, 'Adam just say to Dave, "school boat trip –Christine", and that will shut him up.'

'What happened on the school boat trip?'

'I'm not going to tell you, Adam, but if you want to shut Dave up, just say, "school boat trip – Christine" and he'll think you know all about it and he won't want you talking about it and he'll leave you alone.'

I didn't have much contact with Adam after that. I was far too busy with my own life and business but whenever I saw him or spoke to him on the phone he was happy and confident. I think all it took for Adam to progress was someone to believe in him and for Adam to experience success and once his parents changed their attitude towards him he flourished. We live in a very judgemental world and we judge on appearance, on medical labels and on norms! I judge on individuality, character and personality. I know Adam had overcome immense prejudice to achieve the success he has achieved. I'm afraid Adam's 'disability' is not the medical label he bears but society and individuals in that society. How grateful I am for my parents and my immediate family who believed in me and championed me through the many challenges of my younger years and I'm even more grateful to Kathleen, my wife, for she has supported me and sustained me through the many experiences of our life together.

My business went from strength to strength and I was amazed at where all my work came from. I never advertised. All my work came from recommendations. My only purpose in setting up in business was to support my family. Initially, I didn't know whether it was going to work or not. I used part of my garage as an office because I could not afford to rent other accommodation. We kept our overheads as low as possible. I really had a limited view of the issues around disability and I needed to widen that view if I were to represent other disabled people and their issues in the training room. I looked around for organisations of disabled people and went to meet them. I met people from the local Councils of Disabled People and from the local groups of disabled people. I visited work centres and hostels. I spoke with as many disabled people as I could in order to include the real issues in my work. I came face to face with the national disability movement. These people were aggressive activists who were fighting the establishment. I'm afraid I'm not militant or confrontational and the 'activists' actually scared me. They were willing to chain themselves to buses and railings. They would be part of public demonstrations. They would risk being arrested by the police and the consequences of that. I'm afraid I discovered I was not the kind of person who could demonstrate, etc., but I knew what they were fighting for and I had to find a way of supporting them that suited my character. The least I could do was to represent their issues in the training room. From my dealings with disabled people, I learned about the real issues and I learned about myself. With the knowledge I had gained, I had a basis to improve training programmes and even extend the number and variety of courses I offered.

My client base grew and my work expanded from Disability Equality Training to Personal Development Training. I had commissions for many and varied events. I gained contracts with a number of London Boroughs, with several Central Government Departments and with many Local Authorities. Kathleen came with me and acted as navigator, scribe and personal assistant. It's always been amazing to both of us that many delegates on our training courses have thought Kathleen to be my carer and have commented so and I think, without exception, these comments have come from professional people!

As I gained confidence in what I was doing and as my work yielded enough income to support my home and family, so my interests and orientation changed.

81

I was preoccupied with providing for my family when I began my business but within a few months I developed sincerity of purpose. I felt I could make a difference in many ways through my training courses. I did many courses for Personnel Officers (now Human Resources) these courses contained an equality component but the main orientation was the recruitment and retention of people with disabilities. All the delegates from courses on the recruitment process had to develop an action plan at the end of the course. These were monitored for twelve months after the course and through this process it was discovered that many more disabled people applied for job vacancies, many were successful in being appointed, disabled employees were retained in their jobs and we had evidence of several people who acquired a disability whilst employed and been retrained rather than retired as was the tradition.

Technology is the liberation of many people and I have witnessed miracles through technology. Many are enabled in various areas of life through technology. Many people are able to work because of technology such as speech activation and conversion from the written word to Braille, to name but two! Personally, I have technophobia! I have a very real aversion to technology. I've had so many bad experiences, I now fear technology. My dexterity is such that a keyboard or TV control buttons are my enemy. It is so easy for me to press the wrong key or combinations of keys with disastrous effects. I hate television buttons, DVD players and such and no one understands. When we need to buy a new television I am more interested in the control buttons than anything else. They have to be convenient to my unique dexterity and always my concerns are dismissed and I get angry, really angry, and the people who are with me are embarrassed. Seeking to buy a new television or DVD player is bad enough but having to change my computer is a nightmare! People advise me to go voice-activated. I've tried three times; it doesn't work for me. At the conclusion of every trial with voice activation, I have been told it's because of my speech impediment. Technology scares the daylights out of me. Also, I wonder if it could be something to do with the era I was brought up in. There were no televisions, remote controls or computers when I was younger and so my ideas and values don't centre around technology but around what are now old-fashioned methods of communication. But on training courses I have to present a positive image of technology and I use video and DVD (providing there is someone there to work the machine for me!) to illustrate how liberating and how enabling technology can be in the workplace for disabled people.

I'm very keen on consultation. Although we have improved as a nation in asking disabled people for their views on services and systems which affect them,

I would suggest we have further to go in terms of real individual consultation. There is a need, very often, to train and encourage individuals to speak out and ask for what they want. There has been much progress in many areas of our society in this practice. It was to this end that I was asked to facilitate training courses in personal advocacy. My company was commissioned to design and deliver a training course for one of the London boroughs. One of these courses was for people who had experience of mental illness and the message was that you have a right to ask for what you need or want.

One of the delegates, Jenny, was a wheelchair user who lived in residential accommodation because her husband could no longer manage to care for her at home. Jenny had physical difficulties as well as experience of mental illness. I knew the course had been a success when Jenny shouted to my wife, who was sat in front of the delegates, very publicly from her wheel chair, at a very inappropriate time in the course, 'Nurse, nurse, I want sex with my husband!' The room went silent, there followed embarrassed laughter and two young female care assistants, who had come to the course with Jenny, rushed forward and began removing her from the room.

A very loud 'STOP!' emitted from my throat and the room once again fell into an embarrassed silence.

'Leave her where she is and sit down!' I commanded.

'But-' said one of the care assistants. I interrupted. 'There are no buts. Sit down and I'll deal with this' I've never had such an attentive group as this one while they anticipated what I might do and say next. I walked up the room, stood directly in front of the woman in the wheelchair and spoke to her directly:

'Well done! Can you and I talk in the break?'

The woman beamed a flashing smile and nodded her head and I addressed the group. 'Is this what happens when you speak out and ask for your needs? Do members of staff try to shut you up? Are you oppressed? How do you deal with this kind of thing?' I then turn to Kathleen and I actually don't need to speak. Kathleen whispers, 'I know where you're going with this one. I'll put them into small groups and get them to discuss the questions you've just asked while you talk to Jenny.

As Kathleen takes over the group, I ask Jenny to come with me to a quiet corner of the room where we can talk quietly. I had not noticed before but Jenny could not move her own wheelchair. I had to push her!

Jenny and I settled in a quiet corner of the room away from the rest of the group and we were joined by an uninvited care worker. 'I need to have a quiet and private word with Jenny,' I say.

'I'm her care worker and I am here to look after her'!

'Wonderful' I say, 'But have you asked Jenny if she wants you here? I know your role but you can observe from afar. We are in the same room – unless Jenny wants you to be part of our conversation!' Jenny shook her head and dismissed the care worker in no uncertain terms through her body language.

'Right, Jenny, I haven't much time. Talk to me about your needs.'

Jenny expressed sorrow and apologised for shouting out as she did and added, 'I get so frustrated. I do silly things like that. It's like I panic!'

'It's alright. It doesn't matter. Just talk to me!' I said encouragingly. It didn't take very long for Jenny to tell me she was 52 years of age. She had been the head teacher of a local primary school. She had been diagnosed with multiple sclerosis four years ago, which had progressed quite rapidly, and she had a mental breakdown a year ago. Her husband could not manage to care for her at home and she had been in residential care for nine months. She felt she had lost everything. She expressed that she had a longing for her husband, a need within her that could not be fulfilled in any other way. She said she sat all day in her wheelchair, watched the other residents and thought 'am I like them?' She said, 'If I start to weep, they will come and take me away from you and I want to continue.' So we moved deeper into the corner and tried to become a little more private. Jenny carried on telling me she didn't feel a woman any longer and there was no way her husband wanted her anymore because she was no longer attractive. She longed to snuggle up to her husband, longed for the comfort of the intimacy they used to have together, longed for the assurance that she and her husband still had that special relationship which made her feel a real woman and filled her world. Her husband came to visit her every Saturday and often on a Sunday too. But they didn't have any privacy; they had to visit in the lounge of the residential home with the other residents and visitors around and with the staff constantly coming and going.

I had to cut short the conversation with Jenny because I had to get back to the group but I promised to talk with her at the end of the day if possible.

The whole group was 'buzzing' with comments and ideas about how they could become more assertive and how they might ask for their individual needs and this stemmed from Jenny's earlier outburst. There was however a little pessimism, a lack of confidence that what I was suggesting could ever happen. When I explained that the local authority were actually paying me to do this work – paying travelling expenses, paying for overnight accommodation and paying me a fee – the group concluded that the authority wouldn't pay all that money if they didn't mean it.

At the end of the course each individual had to create an action plan. They actually wrote down a step-by-step plan of how they were going to put into practice what they had learned from the course! I was really surprised that when we had feedback from these action plans, most people had said two things. They wanted another day, specifically with me because I was less threatening than other people and they didn't want care workers sat at the back of the room in their own little group. They thought care workers should join in the training or stay out of the training room.

The action planning session on any course can be hectic as there are always many delegates who seek my help. So I really hadn't time to spend with Jenny. But I needn't have worried because Kathleen was with Jenny. I thought it very telling that we had five care workers sitting at the back of the room but it was Kathleen who had gone to Jenny's aid. Jenny needed someone to write for her! At the end of the day there wasn't time to talk with Jenny because transport had come to take Jenny back to her home. Jenny left with her action plan, which she said would be an enormous help to her.

It was a different Jenny who attended a course with the same group of delegates a month later. This course was so difficult to fit into my diary as it was extra to the commissioned courses which had been planned and booked months ago. This extra course was in response to the delegates' request and it gave credence to the message that the local authority was trying to give. We also had a woman in attendance from Social Services who took control of the care workers.

It was like meeting up with old friends again. The first question I asked the delegates was, 'How are your action plans going?' Jenny was the first to reply and it was incredible to see her so animated. She really had lots of success. I hadn't seen her action plan at the end of the last course but her first piece of action was to question her medication for her mental health problems and this she had done. She was now being weaned off this medication and felt better, and many of the other delegates agreed that although they knew they needed the medication to control their mental health problems, it made them feel much worse. Not having experienced these kinds of problems, I could not give opinion or comment but Jenny had certainly made progress. She had been home at the weekend, just for the daytime, and it was hoped that her home could be adapted to her physical needs so that she might return home permanently. She was also being assessed for an electric wheelchair which she could operate herself and which would give her independence and mobility. Her husband had found the behaviour caused by her mental illness difficult to manage and now that she had recovered, he could cope with the physical issues. Jenny had also been allocated a social worker who was really helpful and was in liaison with other agencies to enable Jenny to return to live in her own home. I would say that being part of the planning process was important to Jenny and helped her recovery somewhat but it can be very difficult to know what one needs in the way of adaptation and aids when one goes through a great personal change. The unexpected happens so seldom, few of us plan for it and know how to deal with it. The majority of us have ordered lives for most of the time. We seem to live within a spectrum of known possibilities, experiences to which we have learned responses. Outside of this spectrum we find chaos, a darker world that we have no experience of and no guidelines for. How do we cope? Jenny's multiple sclerosis was totally unexpected and maybe the effects of the unexpected had caused her to become confused and disorientated as to need the respite provided by drugs. I don't know if Jenny had reasoned things out in her drugged, stupefied mind but she now seemed able to accept the changes to herself and her life and begin to plan and organise for her future.

Lots of the other delegates had success stories to tell too; most of them saw the benefits of 'speaking out' on their own behalf and were planning to become participative rather than passively accepting what others said they should do and have. I enjoyed the feedback and felt really proud that my training could affect the lives of others so positively. It did my reputation no harm, either, to have the woman from Social Services evaluate the course with the delegates at the end of the day.

CHAPTER FIVE

Throughout my previous employment I have dealt with people of all descriptions in many and varied situations. In all of my jobs it's been vital that I have understood people and what motivates each individual. I have also learned the importance of how people react to me. I've always been aware of how many people are put off by my impeded speech, my posture and my appearance. I always make allowances and give people time to get to know me. It's important to me to have the people I'm dealing with feel okay around me – fundamentally they need to see me as a person, not a disability. Otherwise, in my experience, I get nothing out of them.

The world of mainstream employment is a trillion miles away from the world of self-employment but my past experience prepared me for the new adventure of running my own business. In this new and exciting venture, my disability is a key factor, as I present issues experienced by disabled people. I am a visual, real-life example and really I haven't time to allow people to see past my speech impediment –often I meet potential clients by talking to them on the phone, which is not my best method of communication. I experienced a lot of rejection. I heard many negatives: 'How could you ever deliver training with your speech?' or, 'it's a bit early in the day for drinking isn't it?' and many more much worse comments. I had to battle with the effect these comments had on me. They took me back to earlier experiences in my younger years. I could not allow my confidence to be affected. I really had to believe in myself. I was motivated by having to pay a mortgage and support a wife and family. As, eventually and fortunately for me, most of my work came from other people's recommendation, I had no need to advertise or participate in cold selling on the phone.

When you put people in front of a 'disabled' trainer they feel uncomfortable and self-conscious. An essential part of my job as a facilitator is to put people at their ease. I like to speak to as many delegates as I can before the start of a training course and spend the first half hour or so saying very little of importance so that people have the time and ability to tune into my speech and adjust their attitudes to my appearance and unique body language.

My previous life taught me self-discipline and how to be organised. I pride myself on being professional and beginning and ending on time. I am always well-prepared, for I have learned from sore experience of the past that to fail to prepare is to prepare for a failure.

A great deal of work has gone into achieving the reputation I have. I feel my life experiences have prepared me as a trainer in my chosen field. I feel a great responsibility as a trainer, for I represent others, like me, who bear the label 'disabled person' and maybe, just maybe, hopefully I am affecting the future of many as I work with Human Resource personnel, large employers and service providers.

I am ever-conscious of my appearance and how many react to my impeded speech and my uncontrollable facial movements. My hand function is awkward and some people react to my unusual handshake. My dexterity, too, is unique and becomes very obvious when I distribute handouts or shuffle papers. I also experience a painful spasm which causes unusual twitches in my body. I use eye contact to compensate for these peculiarities, I need to allow people to get to know me and see past my disability, and through eye contact I can express sincerity, self-belief, intelligence and an 'it's alright to be me' aura. I also use humour to put people at their ease and do have a twinkle in my eye too. My appearance is important, for through it I can powerfully illustrate many of the issues I'm presenting.

I am a self-confessed people watcher and learn a lot from this. Usually I know which people are most affected by my disability and I make sure I chat to them before I begin training. I can usually spot someone, too, who will respond effectively to my sense of humour. Although my training is very intense and serious, and often heavy, I know from experience that laughter lightens the atmosphere and helps the learning process – a spoonful of sugar…

Throughout my married life, my aim has been to provide for my wife and adorable children. I'm not sure I've been ambitious beyond this. I think having been told that I would never work when I was younger has made me value my employment and has created a real fear of losing my job. Often I have been told that it would be easier for me if I lived on state benefits. But somehow I have avoided this and I value my work ethos, and every training course I am commissioned to undertake is really important to me and every commissioning client receives my utmost attention. Maybe I am incredibly pragmatic and forward thinking. I have to be aware of my competitors in business and I am always keen to expand and develop my repertoire in offering training.

It took me many years to accept who I am and what I am and I have suffered from constant messages from many sources which implanted negativity about being me! It is so easy to compare myself to others but through time I have accepted my identity. I like being me and it's the comparisons that have caused the damage in the past. I now refuse to even think of comparing myself to others. I am uniquely individual and proud of it. Rising above the low expectations of my early life has given me immense pleasure.

When I began Focus disABILITY in the late 1980s, it was a time of great change as we were entering the EEC and becoming involved in social charters, and anti-discriminatory legislation had a high profile in the disability movement and on political agendas. All of this had an effect on the interest in disability throughout society.

More and more disabled people were challenging society and were refusing to accept the traditional care, cure and charity approach. They were demanding choices and rights on a scale never before experienced in history. These demands were not extra to other people's demands: they were basic human rights, principally – equal opportunities in employment.

Most non-disabled people had a narrow thinking on disability. They limited the issues to wheelchair users or blind or deaf. They didn't think beyond these well-known disabilities unless they had personal experience through a family member or close friend. In general, people attending my training courses needed to be aware of the extensive variety of disability – wheelchair users, people who have difficulty with movement, deafness, blindness, people with learning difficulties, people with mental health problems, language and speech problems, hidden disability such as asthma, epilepsy, heart conditions, diabetes… The list is endless and we needed to extend it to include congenital and acquired disability.

Training was necessary to reveal the attitudes of people in our society towards those of us with disabilities. It was becoming increasingly obvious that inaccessible environments and tradition caused disability rather than whatever label or medical diagnosis may be attached to a person. The very fabric of our society caused so many problems for so many people. For example, if a person is unable to walk then they are provided with a wheelchair. A wheelchair is given to enable, not to disable. There are thousands of wheelchair users who are very able to propel and manoeuvre their wheelchairs very skilfully and efficiently – until they encounter steps, stairs, narrow doorways, etc. The person's ability has not changed – it's the prohibitions caused by society which are the problem. Many people could apply for jobs if the application form were in the correct format and relevant to individuals, and many people might be more successful at interview if the interviewing panel were aware of their own personal attitudes!

The Disabled Persons (Employment) Acts of 1944 and 1958 regarded 'people with disabilities' to be those people who have a disability that interferes with their capacity to obtain or keep employment which, aside from that disability, would normally be suited to their age, experience and qualification. For all employers who employed over twenty people, these acts made it a legal requirement for at least three per cent of their workforce to be registered disabled people. Of course, it was very easy for many employers to gain exemption from this percentage and the legislation was not enforceable anyway. So discrimination was widespread and had not really been addressed.

I discovered a survey carried out in 1988, the year I became ill, and started researching and thinking of my own business. This survey by the OPCS identified 6.2 million disabled people in Great Britain; this was considered to be on the low side by the disability movement as it was known that many people with disability did not participate in the survey because, it was said, the design of the questionnaire was offensive to them. So, maybe, disability involved a larger proportion of our society than was reported.

It seemed to me that the traditional recruitment process was full of barriers that affected a vast number of people. Many companies were proud of their 'equal opportunity policy' but oblivious to the discrimination caused through their recruitment practices.

Most people were introduced to their current jobs through a job advertisement in a newspaper or a professional magazine. I researched hundreds of job advertisements and found most of them unfriendly and off-putting to disabled people. Traditionally, the employment market had not included disabled people and in my training programmes I suggested that unless advertisements effectively targeted and positively encouraged people with disabilities, they would not apply. I was aware through talking with a variety of disabled people that frequent rejection in the past had discouraged them and destroyed their confidence.

I developed a clientele of companies who employed large numbers of people. These companies were interested in employing disabled people but didn't seem to attract applications for their job vacancies from people who had disabilities. As I became more confident in my ability to train, assess the training needs of these companies and create training programmes, so I became more challenging. I nurtured a good, sound working relationship with training managers and chief personnel officers and always discussed with them the findings of my research into their companies training needs and how I was going to address those needs in the training room. Many of my methods were very unconventional and controversial and many times I was told 'You can't do that!' But I knew that I could. I used my sense of humour and my personality. I developed a relationship with each delegate who attended my courses. I limited the number of delegates on each course to twelve people so that I could manage to be personally involved with each delegate and be sensitive to their feelings, particularly as they became challenged by some of my presentations and training exercises. The issues involved were rather heavy and the content of a training course challenged delegates' personal and individual attitudes. Training also challenged tradition and practices, and I know many felt guilty when issues were introduced to them and part of my role as a facilitator was to 'comfort', 'placate' and help people use their guilt towards positive outcomes. Those outcomes meant that people with disability who were unemployed might find work easier to access. Certainly the research I did revealed that the companies I had worked for were changing their policies and practices through my training and were attracting and recruiting disabled people.   I was paid to do a job. I also had competitors and I needed to do a good job, earn my fee and gain good evaluations and outcomes so that the companies I worked for would always come to me to supply their training needs, rather than go to my competitors!

One of my exercises was really devious but always had a profound effect. I would look at the companies' current job vacancies, select a few appointments and with the help of a chief personnel officer, and using fictional names, I would send in a model application with a letter as well. Then I would send in the same application but introduce a disability. Always, my 'non-disabled' applications would be invited to interview but applications declaring disabilities were never shortlisted. There were very sensitive issues involved in this and I was not able to present the actual applications on all courses because my relationship with the group had to be right and sometimes a group didn't gel too well. But, on some courses, where I felt comfortable, I presented both applications as a training exercise and delegates were terribly shocked at the revelation. Sometimes the person who had signed the rejection letters before they were sent out would be a delegate on the course but their signature was removed from the letter before it was presented to the delegates.

Sometimes delegates would have helped sieve and shortlist. Initially, the training room would go quiet as these application forms were presented and people wanted to justify their part in this outcome but I was skilful in diverting these comments and distracting delegates from justifying themselves into looking at the real issues involved.

The discussion following this exercise was always revealing! The delegates would be directed to discuss why people worked – disability did not come into this discussion. Then there was discussion on what each delegate would need to do their present job should they acquire a specific disability. The outcome was usually quite astounding as delegates discovered that the majority of jobs could be done by disabled people, incurring very small financial cost. The discussion always flowed into delegates recognising their own individual and personal attitudes and recognising real discrimination.

At the end of every course, I demanded that each person attending the course design an individual action plan. I always insisted that 'action planning' was written into my contract before I accepted a commission to facilitate any training. My contract would always identify a specifically named person working in the company who would check up on action from each delegate's plan at least every month for a year. The outcomes from many action plans were often tremendous in their impact on policy and practice. One company, for example, recruited a woman who was deaf and used British Sign Language. Before too long, two of her hearing colleagues who worked nearby were attending classes to learn British Sign Language outside of work time. At the end of a year, when I checked on the outcome of action planning, I was told that the company now employed five people who used British Sign Language as their method of communication and many staff had learned or were learning British Sign Language. Another spinoff from this was that it had been noticed that the staff of the department where these five deaf people worked had become more caring towards each other and the atmosphere had changed. I had the opportunity to question a few members of staff from this department who readily told me that they felt secure working for a company who employed disabled people because they felt the company had become more caring and they felt that, should they acquire a disability whilst working for the company, they would be looked after! Certainly, it was obvious to me as I spoke with the managing director that company policy was changing, for they no longer retired employees who acquired disability but tried to retain or retrain them!

I could never say I was a confident person. I think I ignored my shyness, for I knew that holding back would not bring in any work contracts and so I just had to go for it and 'pretend' to be 'confident'. Witnessing the changes that were happening in some of the companies I worked for gave me a real buzz and made me pinch myself to make sure I wasn't dreaming! Success may breed success but for me success bred confidence!

There are times when I work alongside other trainers with disabilities. These time are of real value to me as my methods and abilities as a trainer and the content of my programme were evaluated, albeit informally, by other people who had experience of disability, undoubtedly different to mine, but they had knowledgeable experience of the relevant issues.

I met Chris through a training we did together and we got on like a house on fire. Our friendship blossomed and we spent time together whenever we could. Through this friendship I realised how much I had changed! In the past I would shun disabled people and never associate with them on a social level, maybe because I didn't want to be identified with them. Now I was aware of how wrong I was and how restrictive my attitudes were. What an idiot I was in the past — today some of the best people I know have disabilities and the most amazing people I know, who have become my best friends are classed by the authorities of our country as disabled people. All of these people have so much to offer and my life is totally enhanced by their friendship. I dread to think of all I missed out on in the past because of my attitudes!

Training had become very important to me. Every individual who attended one of my training courses were special to me. I suppose my teacher training came into play. I viewed each delegate as an individual and quickly assessed their level of awareness in relation to the programme of the day. Some delegates were like empty vessels devoid of awareness and I had the challenge to fill this void with knowledge and an awareness which would stimulate personal and corporate changes which would benefit and raise opportunities for disabled people. One of the most important aims on almost every course I facilitated was to challenge and develop an awareness of personal attitudes. I believe attitudes govern behaviour and behaviour governs our relationships with others. The right attitudes affect company and corporate policies which in turn affect the employment and lives of disabled people.

The work Chris and me did together was intense and we needed a diversion after a day in the training room. Neither of us drank., so we found relaxation in humour and just sharing the same world. We were able to communicate together in our own way and we both found it liberating to be in each other's company.

Chris and I developed a reputation amongst our friends. We were named as the terrible twins. Whenever we were together, apart from when we were working in the training room, there would be laughter. Although we also used controlled humour in the training room!   It was part of our relationship; we bounced off each other. We just had this innate ability to make each other, and the people around us, laugh. Was it Mark Twain who said, 'The human race has only one really effective weapon, and that is laughter! The moment it arises, all your irritations and resentments slip away and the sunny spirit takes their place.' Chris and I were very aware of the ignorance, the prejudice and the fear that greeted us every day and when we were together, our remedy to combat the effects of the negatives we experienced from others was humour and an ability to laugh at ourselves.

Maybe I had been working for myself for eighteen months or so when I received a call from the personnel office of a large pharmaceutical company who were interested in my services. As I visited with a representative, I became aware of the potential within this company for work for disabled people and lots of training courses for me to lead. I really wanted to impress and gain the contract on offer. I suppose this meeting was a turning point for me as I became aware that I was a skilled communicator. I had a personality. I had the ability to discuss issues and to win people over. I did not dwell on my impediment or my disability but I became positive in a way I hadn't felt before. At this time in my life I questioned what I was about. Yes, supporting my home and my family was the major priority. But also my business was about improving the lives of others. The long-term aim of my company is to work with employers to provide whatever is needed to give disabled people choice, empowerment and freedom to work in mainstream employment with support if necessary, provided appropriate to individual need. From my experience, employment is an antidote for anxiety: it builds confidence and character. Work is an ointment for sorrow and a doorway to possibility and development. Whatever our circumstances in life, I believe we should all have the same equal right to earn our living through gainful employment. On the other hand, I also believe that people have an equal right not to work, relevant to their personal circumstances. I have lived with my problems all of my life and I had learned and developed skills. For me, through the experience of employment, I had produced a great work in living and achieving. I had a success story to share and I was very proud of my accomplishments. Why then did I shrivel and feel inadequate when faced by others, particularly those who could offer me contracts for future work? My training came from a journey of understanding: throughout my life I had to come to terms with who and what I am. That journey gave me the opportunity to fully explore a whole range of issues. It gave me space to make sense of my feelings and, most importantly, it has focused my attention and given me the means to take action and do positive things for myself, my wife, my family and other people. I have everything in life I could wish for: a supportive, loving and compatible wife, three adorable children, a comfortable home and a means of earning an income. Through my training I want to communicate. I want people who haven't a disability to know what it feels like for those who have. I want my journey to provide a talking point for others – acting as a kick start so that the issues can be brought out in the open and discussed honestly.

I had a determined feeling as I spoke with the man from the pharmaceutical company and I must have impressed him as I was offered the contract there and then. I was further surprised when I was told that references were not needed as I had come highly recommended.

On the second course for recruitment personnel from this pharmaceutical company, I encountered a man who I named 'Mr Odd Bod'. I had twelve delegates on this particular course; well… eleven delegates and Mr Odd Bod! He separated himself from the main group and his participation in the course was minimal. I was concerned. The delegates were all professional people and I'm sure they dressed accordingly when in the office. On a training day, however, they wore casual clothing. Not Mr Odd Bod! He attended the course each day immaculately dressed, booted and suited. I did not know his designation in the company and as he didn't participate, it was difficult for me to assess if he was gaining anything from the two-day course. I found him rather intimidating! As I encouraged him to join in small group activities and to answer questions in whole group activities and discussions, he offered very little and didn't mix with the others. He appeared to be a loner! As I tried to engage him and integrate him with the others in the group, his responses made me question who he was and why he was there. He seemed to be patronising me – and yet I could not be sure. He did have a superior air and attitude about him.

It was during the final session of the course, whilst all the other delegates were involved in creating their action plans, that I had to challenge Mr Odd Bod, for whilst everyone else was focused and talking to each other, he just sat alone, seemingly gazing into space. I approached him and explained that he had to do an action plan; it was a compulsory element of the course. His reaction to this was to say, rather aggressively I thought, 'My action plan is in my head. It is. I want to see you in my office tomorrow morning!' Tomorrow was my rest day and the company was at least eighty miles from my home. I explained and he replied, 'I'm aware of where you live and I will pay for a hotel tonight and I will pay you a day's training fee if you can be in my office tomorrow morning at ten!' I couldn't refuse. Mr Odd Bod turned out to be the managing director of the company and he was so impressed and very complimentary by the way I had facilitated the training course he had attended. His comments did much for my ego. But the main purpose for asking me to meet with him was to ask if I could find a disabled person to fill a future vacancy within the company. This vacancy was for a senior management position. The vacancy was due to the future retirement of the person in post. This person could retire in four months' time but had agreed to stay in post until a suitable person could be found as his successor. I really wasn't sure that I knew of any one suitably qualified for the post but promised to look around.

CHAPTER SIX

I suppose it's inevitable when one runs a business from home that one's leisure time is interrupted by telephone calls. We did have an answer phone but we also had teenagers in our family and they could not allow the phone to ring and not answer it. After all, it might be for them!!!

So reluctantly, I left the work I was doing in the garden and took a phone call, which my lovely daughter had answered. I was somewhat disgruntled at being disturbed because it was mid-March and the first time in the year I had been able to get out in the garden to tidy it up after the winter.

Picking up the phone, I spoke a very curt 'Hello,' and a woman answered and gabbled at me. 'I know you can help my son. Will you come and see him?' I didn't know how to respond. I wanted to get back to my garden and there was a moment's awkward silence as the woman waited for my response. After a long pause, the woman spoke again, rather agitatedly, I thought:

'You're my last hope. Every one says you can help him. Please come.'

The pleading in her voice, mixed with the anguish, softened my mood and got my attention.

I really cannot turn down a person in need.

Her son had married four years ago and went on honeymoon to Spain. He jumped into the swimming pool on a dark night at a very late hour at the hotel where he was staying with his new wife, and injured his spine because there was no water in the pool. He was now a wheelchair user. He was eventually airlifted to England and spent ten months in hospital. His mum and dad had visited him whilst he was in hospital but he refused to see them after he had left hospital. It was obvious to me as mum spoke on the phone that she was heartbroken at not being able to see her son. He was living with his wife at his

97

mother-in-law's home! What could I do? Why me? The guy may not want anything to do with me anyway! Mother was insistent that she knew I could help. Well! I wasn't very comfortable but I said I would meet the guy if he was agreeable. His name was Gordon and I was to phone Sheila, his wife, to arrange my visit. Sheila knew that mum had phoned me.

So, with some trepidation I phoned Sheila to arrange my visit, explaining that I wasn't sure how I could help. I was rather surprised to discover that Gordon lived ninety miles from my home! Why hadn't I asked where they lived before I said I would go? Although business was doing well, we didn't know what the future held and as a family we lived very frugally. So the cost of doing a hundred and eighty-mile round trip was a concern. I was further concerned because Sheila had said that Gordon may not see me anyway. My visit was going to be a surprise to him! Were they to tell him beforehand, he would definitely not see me. Was I going to waste time and money by travelling one hundred and eighty miles on an unproductive and wasted trip?

On the arranged day I arrived at Gordon's home and was welcomed by Sheila's mum. Although the actual building seemed rather old, the room I was shown into had a large bay window and was light and airy, very clean, tidy and well-decorated and furnished. A rather comfortable room, I thought. As is the custom, I was offered a drink of tea. I don't drink tea anyway but I do have problems drinking! My hand function is such that I can't hold a drinking vessel; it has to be placed on a surface in front of me and the ergonomics have to be right or I'm likely to get more liquid down the outside of me than the inside. So I declined the offer of a drink! Sheila wasn't home; she was at work, so mum and I chatted for a little while and I learned mum was a widow and had a part time cleaning job. She worked early in the morning before Sheila left the house for work and in the evening after Sheila returned from work. This was so that Gordon was never alone. I did wonder where Gordon was and I explained how anxious I was about meeting him. I was told he lived in the back room and never came out of that room. It was then explained to me that he was in a good mood that day.

Eventually, mum opened the door from the room we were in to the back room. The smell which emanated was a surprise to me!

Mum said rather hesitatingly and timidly, 'Gordon, there's a man here to see you!'

The reply was, 'Don't want to see no man. Tell him to f…. off!'

Mum's rather embarrassed reply was, 'Oh Gordon, don't be like that. The

98

man's here now. He's come a long way to see you. Please be nice.'

'I don't want to see anyone. I bet he's another bloody social worker or a f***ing do-gooder. I'm sick of them. Just go away and leave me alone.'

Mum and I stood just outside the door to Gordon's room during this interchange and I gulped in my throat and had to look away from the eyes which were appealingly looking into mine, communicating a fearful aura of 'I don't know what to do'. I could feel the panic in this woman and I wondered what other language might be hurled from behind the door. I knew that she was feeling embarrassed on my behalf. I put my hand on her arm to indicate I was fine and I shouted through the door, 'Gordon. My name is Alan. I am neither a social worker nor a do-gooder. Like you, I've had a bellyful of them. I don't know why I'm here. Your mother rang me and asked if I would meet you. I can go away right now if you want me to, but I won't come back and I don't like talking to a door!'

Instantly, Gordon replied, 'You sound different, like you might know what you're talking about. Come in.'

Mum ushered me through the door with great relief and enthusiasm.

Gordon's appearance was a shock to me. He was unshaven. His hair looked uncombed and dishevelled; it seemed to have been chopped by an amateur rather than cut by a professional. His clothes were dirty and scruffy and his whole appearance left a lot to be desired. He was slumped rather than sat in a wheel chair and I could not recognise or describe the putrid smell which permeated the room. There was a window in the room which overlooked a conservatory. It appeared to me that this conservatory had been turned into a dining room to house Gordon in what was the original dining room.

Gordon's room was dingy, to say the least. It housed a single bed, a chair, which turned out to be a commode, a wardrobe, a music centre and a small portable television and that was all. The bed covering looked clean and matched the curtains at the window.

Gordon offered me his hand and looked a little shocked when I refused it and explained about my poor hand function. He invited me to sit down and I chose to sit on the edge of the bed because I was suspicious of what the commode might contain.

I began the conversation by telling him about his mother's phone call. Gordon ignored this and answered by asking me what was wrong with me.

Usually, I respond to this kind of question quite rudely, for I don't consider there to be anything 'wrong' with me, and my medical details are private. My stock answer to 'what's wrong with you?' is, 'You tell me about your sex life and I'll tell you what's wrong with me.' No one has ever told me about their sex life and I have not told too many people what's wrong with me! My philosophy on this is that I am a person first and foremost and I want to be accepted as a person. I do not want to be a phenomenon of any kind; neither do people understand medical labels. If I need to justify my existence by explaining what's 'wrong' then I don't want to play.

Of course, it's different with Gordon: if I was going to be of any help to him, I needed to develop a relationship with him and being rude or political might deter this.

I explained all about myself in detail so that he knew that maybe my problems were not as trivial as he might think.

I then asked him about himself and listened with sympathy to a tirade of awful language and tales of woe. His voice was almost breaking, as if he were on the verge of tears, as he related the details of his accident and his treatment in hospital. He told me about his traumatic experiences with therapists and social workers and I really felt for him. Not a word did he say about how all that had happened to him affected his wife or parents or indeed his mother-in-law. His conversation was all me, me, me and interlaced with the foulest of language. This man was so bitter! I knew the hospital where he had been treated and they have a really good reputation in every field, but they excel in the area of rehabilitation. Although Gordon had been away from the hospital for about three years, I could not imagine him being discharged from hospital in the negative state he was in to live in this highly inappropriate and inconvenient accommodation. And I asked, 'Were you discharged from hospital or did you discharge yourself?' My assumption was right; he had discharged himself! He was hurting and the hurt made him bitter, angry and very selfish. Maybe I can identify with Gordon's state of mind. I think we all have scars. Not necessarily from an accident but the scars of a painful past. Some of those scars are unsightly and have caused hurt and deep regret but life is for living and in the struggle to live a meaningful life with our scars there is personal growth and development. There was a lot I didn't agree with in Gordon's account of events and happenings but I tried to avoid any confrontation. Gordon had not been neglected by his local authority. They had sent in care workers; he had a social worker and a physiotherapist attend him at home but he had dismissed them as interfering busybodies and refused to have them in his room. He had attended a number of day and work centres but after a few weeks had refused to go because he didn't like the other people who attended. He had a few mates from his past who had invited him to go with them to the pub but he had declined. He and his wife had been offered an adapted bungalow in the past but Gordon had turned it down and chose to live with his mother-in-law because he said there was a stigma to living in a council property and everyone knew that the particular bungalow had been adapted. I didn't quite understand his reasoning on the housing issue and I was reluctant to challenge but I did explained that his life could be improved if he could listen to a social worker and a physiotherapist. Secretly, I was thinking; if all these people have failed to help him – then what am I doing here?

I mentioned his parents and he became very agitated and foulmouthed. I thought again that he was going to cry! The thoughts that Gordon expressed about his feelings towards his parents were so intense as to affect me emotionally. Gordon reacted to my tears with complete amazement and asked why I was crying. 'Gordon,' I said, 'There is nothing wrong in crying. I am crying because of what has happened to you and because of this (indicating the room) and because of your parents.' There was a silent pause and he just sat staring at me as though I had two heads. 'Gordon,' I said 'I am a parent and if my son ever said to me that he didn't want to see me again for whatever reason, I would be absolutely devastated!'

Gordon's face registered deep thoughtfulness and I anticipated that he was thinking about the situation between him and his parents. I was quite wrong! He exclaimed, in shocked tones, 'What do you mean you're a parent? You have kids!?'

'Yes. I have three children, one son and two daughters. I have a wife as well!'

'What do you mean you have three kids? Are they really yours or are they adopted?'

This assumption and ignorance would normally infuriate me and I would aggressively attack the attitudes that created such comments. Gordon was not the first to question my manhood but I allowed him to get away with it and calmly told him that my children were mine. They were not adopted. I was their natural father. His next remark also annoyed me:

'What's your wife like? Is she disabled too?'

I am sure my annoyance showed on my face, but I answered calmly, 'No, my wife is not disabled and before you ask, my children are not disabled either!' I could almost hear the cogs working in his head as he thought about this revelation. I gave him a little time to think but didn't allow any more questions. I intercepted his verbal reaction by assertively stating, 'Right, young man, I'm going to say one more thing about me and we will move on to talk about you. Is that okay?' Gordon nodded and I continued, 'I was born the way I am and I've had lots of time to get used to being me. I like who I am and I do not want to be normal. To become normal would mean I would have to change and that change would be really difficult. I wouldn't cope! I can't be made better anyway so I've got to accept who I am and make the best of it.'

After thinking for a while, he looked like he had been struck by lightning and talked and talked and talked. I just sat and listened. The most important statement he made was, 'I don't want anyone to see me as I am, least of all my parents. I realise I'm hiding myself away. How can you say you like who you are?' I reacted with empathy:

'I absolutely know what you are saying. I've had this conversation with myself many times. But ask yourself why you don't want to be you. It's because of what others might think, say or do. I decided long ago that this is my life and it's got nothing to do with anyone else. I've only got one life. I'm going to make the most of it. Bugger the rest!'

I paused for breath, he looked at me wide-eyed and I continued:

'What should I do, Gordon? Look at me. I'm disabled. I am not like other people. I can't speak properly. Should I shut myself away and become a pathetic disabled person and not even try to communicate with people or should I grab life with both hands and enjoy living it my way? Gordon, I don't care what others think about me. Bugger them. It's what I think about myself!'

This really got Gordon fired up and again he talked. He spoke about his past life; how active he had been and how popular he had been with his mates and with the ladies. He talked about the fears he had of facing life as a disabled person and he told me about the way he relived his accident every night in his sleep. He talked about all the perceived negatives of his new identity.

I did not know how to respond. I felt completely out of my depth. I muttered more, then said, 'Gordon, I don't know what to say or how I can help. I came here because your mum called me!'

He looked at me with a look of amazement on his face and in rapid tones replied, 'But you've already helped. Although it's embarrassing, I'd like to tell you something! I heard your voice through the door and I thought "Let him in. Let's have a laugh!" I wondered what the bloody hell it was coming to visit me. You walked into this room and I did not expect to see what I saw. I know now that I judged you from the sound of your voice and I was so surprised at your appearance. You look so smart. The way you've talked to me, you have made me feel inferior and really awful; I'm just wasting my life!'

To say I was dumbfounded is an understatement and there was a very embarrassed silence. He broke the silence by saying, 'I've met other disabled people, in the hospital and at various centres I've been to and they all seem to be plonkers. I've never met anyone I could get on with but you're different.' I recovered my composure and told him that my main reason for coming was his mum. I asked what he would say to his mum if she were here. His mood seemed to change and he looked challenged and said, 'Well, mum would not be here!'

'Gordon, I don't understand. Why won't you see your mum? Don't answer that. Don't think about it. I'm going to ask again and you are going to say the first thing that comes into your head. Ready? ... No hesitation. Just tell me, why won't you see your mum?' I received an instant reply, 'Because I'm embarrassed because I've let her down.'

'How have you let her down?'

'Because I can never be the son she wants me to be. I know she had great expectation of me and now I'm stuck like this and I can't be what she expects me to be!'

There followed a long conversation, mostly on blame. Gordon confessed he blamed himself for his accident – after all, he had jumped in the empty pool! The conversation went on and on.

I was with him for ages and the time came for me to leave. I was most surprised when Gordon asked if I would visit him again. I said I would on certain conditions:

A. That he aired his room and got rid of the awful smell.

B. He smartened himself up in dress and grooming.

C. He completed the homework that I was about to give him.

These forthright requests brought a tirade of justifications. He confessed that he was not fussy about emptying his bags. He was doubly incontinent and he had been taught how to look after himself before he was allowed home from hospital but he couldn't be bothered. I explained that I was not going to sit with the smell, particularly if it could be avoided. If he couldn't be bothered to look after himself then neither could I be bothered to see him.

No promises were made but he looked rather sheepish and asked what the home work was. 'Well Gordon.' I said, 'It won't be easy and I want you to get your wife to help you!'

Gordon stopped me in mid-sentence:

'My wife won't help. We hardly speak. She can't stand to be in the same room as me!'

'Gordon!' said I, 'I don't blame Sheila. I have to say this. This room stinks. You also smell. You don't realise the awful smell because you're in it all the time. I'm sorry, I'm being really blunt and I feel I'm being really rude. But if I'm coming to see you again I need to be honest with you.' He looked quite embarrassed and I felt embarrassed but I felt he needed to know. Eventually, Gordon asked about the homework!

'Before I come again, I want you to write a list of at least twenty-four things which are good about you and before you say you can't, let me start your list. You are good looking, you have intelligence. I know this because of the way you've talked today. Behind the hard façade you portray, I am sure there is an attractive personality and I observe you can use your hands really well too. Now you add to the list and I want twenty-four things which are good about you! Get Sheila to help' He nodded at me, half accepting my challenge.

I arose to leave but Gordon said, 'Tell me. When can you come again?' My reply was, 'I don't know. I think my diary is in my car. I'll go and get it and come right back.' Gordon's eyes became like saucers and with surprise in his voice he asked, 'You have a car? You drive a car?'

'Yes, Gordon, I drive a car!'

As I walked through to my car, Sheila's mum met me with a look of surprised anticipation on her face and declared in whispered tones, 'You've been in there a long time. He doesn't usually talk to any one that long.' I didn't have time to reply; Gordon's voice came from the back room: 'You nosey old bat. Keep it out!'

Mum simply put her hands over her mouth and hunched her shoulders and I went to get my diary.

Looking at my diary, I discovered I could visit Gordon again in fifteen days' time and he was delighted with this arrangement. I asked permission to speak bluntly and he said I could.

'Well, Gordon, I need to get something off my chest and it may seem very rude but I'm going to say it anyway. I don't like the way you speak to your mother-in-law. I get the feeling she is frightened of you and it really isn't on. This is her home and she's lost half of it to you. You repay her by calling her an old bat and use bad language and embarrass her in her own home. It's not on. Really, it's not is it?'

I did experience a feeling of fear before I challenged him in this way and as I was awaiting his reply I was feeling really scared. However, he looked at me thoughtfully and held out his hand to me. I took his hand in my left hand and he looked me in the face and said, 'I like you. You've got real guts and every time you open your mouth you make me think.'

'Well, I'm glad I make you think. Relationships are important to me and I actually need people to help me in many different ways and I think you are in the same boat as me. There was a time when maybe I was a tyrant to my mum in particular and she took it because she felt sorry for me and didn't know how to help me. She could not do anything right for me; I was rude, aggressive and really awkward. I knew she was being really kind to me and I also knew I needed her. No way could I manage without her. But at the time, I was hurting. I could see all my peers working and courting and getting married – doing all kinds of things I thought I'd never do. I felt I was being left behind. And now when I look back, I made my mum's life a hell. I was so demanding and domineering. I had a devastating effect on my mum and my family and why, because I was so selfish!'

I could see I'd hit a chord and he was thinking about it. It was obvious he wasn't sure whether I was getting at him or not and he looked at me questionably and asked, 'Are you saying I'm a tyrant and I'm selfish?'

'I'm just relating my experience, that's all.'

'That's all; you say that as though you mean "if the cap fits, wear it".'

I took my leave of Gordon and as I walked through the front room and mother arose from her chair to see me out, I heard Gordon shout, 'Thank you for coming!' At this there was a sharp intake of breath from mum and as I left her on the door step, she exclaimed, 'What have you done to him? He doesn't usually say thank you to anyone for anything. Wait till I tell our Sheila!'

This kind of encounter has a real effect on me. I find it emotionally draining and physically exhausting. I needed to clear my mind of the awful circumstances that Gordon related to me so that I could concentrate on my driving and be safe on the road. I moved my car from the front of Gordon's house and found a quiet layby. I hoped I could nap a while but my mind was full of Gordon. The questions for me were, 'Have I done any good today?' 'Did my visit benefit Gordon in any way?' and 'Would it be worthwhile going back for a second visit?' It would be easy to cancel the arrangement I had made to visit in a few days time! After some deep thinking, I decided I had already made a difference to Gordon's life and I felt that my continued association with him would really help him. I felt a deep assurance that this was so! I cannot say where that assurance came from. I do have a lot of experience of being involved with other people and their problems and I also have intuition! I can't explain what I mean by intuition! It's difficult to describe how it works. For me it's about listening to my own feelings and it's about assessing the feelings others engender in me. I suppose it's a gut feeling, the experience of interpretation of those gut feelings and learning to trust and have confidence in those feelings.

That was it! I'd made a decision! I decided that may be I could help Gordon and I would visit again. I'd made up my mind. I'd cleared my thinking and I could move on. The experience of meeting Gordon and all of his problems were filed away in my mind and I could concentrate and enjoy my drive home.

WOW. I was not prepared for my second visit. Gordon was like a different man! Mum met me at the door with a beaming smile and could not wait to usher me into the house, and welcomed me by saying, 'I'm glad you're here! My name is Enid, by the way!' and turning her head to the door of Gordon's room she shouted, 'Hey buggerlugs! Alan's here, can I tell him what's going on?' The reply was, 'With a gob as big as yours, no one could stop you! But come in here and do it!' This interchange contained humour and Enid laughed. She appeared for more relaxed than on my first visit and the fear in her countenance which I detected on that visit had gone! There was a very different atmosphere in the house. I was ushered into the back room and I braced myself in readiness for the stench. As I entered the room, I was somewhat shocked; what little smell might have remained was masked by a sweet smelling room freshener and Gordon wasn't in the room either. The window was open, as were the double doors of the conservatory, to allow the room to have a current of fresh air. Enid had this smile on her face and I think she was enjoying the surprised expression on my face. She expressed with glee, 'Different, isn't it, but you haven't seen anything yet. He's in the kitchen, go on through.' As I entered the large gleaming kitchen, there was Gordon, sat at a round table with a polished beech wood top on a dining chair, with his folded wheelchair nearby. He greeted me with enthusiasm and a smile! I had been with him for over four hours on my first visit and he hadn't smiled once. He wore a blue shirt that looked freshly laundered and grey trousers. He was freshly shaved, his hair had been combed and his appearance was altogether different than the first time I met him. I spoke to him and I'm sure astonishment manifested in my voice as I said, 'You look really good! What happened?'

Enid and Gordon were obviously excited and both of them wanted to tell me what had happened; they both spoke at once. My 'Whoa, whoa. One at once!' caused them both to go quiet. And they spoke again at the same time and in unison and then they looked at each other, had a little giggle and Gordon put his hand in the air as though halting traffic and said jovially to Enid, 'I surrender. Alright, you win. I can't compete with you when it comes to talking!' Enid smiled at him and then went quiet as though being given permission to speak had somehow stopped her mouth.

'Come, Enid,' I said, 'I want to know, what's happened?'

Enid took a deep breath and started talking:

'Well after you'd gone the last time he called me to him and asked if I was frightened of him and was he a tyrant.'

Immediately I felt guilty because I knew I had put these ideas into his head on my last visit. Enid continued, 'I knew I should be honest with him and I said yes I was frightened of him and he was a tyrant. And we talked about the situation and he said he was going to change and changed he has!' Enid stopped for breath and then continued.

'He moped about in his room after our talk until Sheila came home and he couldn't wait to talk with Sheila. When I came home from work he was tucked up in bed and Sheila was waiting for me and she looked happier than she has looked for years. Sheila's got the afternoon off so she can meet you. She'll be home about 1:30, so I hope you're still here then.'

It was as though someone had wound up Enid and Gordon. I couldn't get a word in edgeways.

Gordon banged on the table and said, 'Could I make coffee now?'

I was trying to say I didn't drink tea or coffee but Enid talked over me, saying,

'See what I mean? He's never made coffee in this house all the time he's lived here. Suddenly, yesterday he decided if we moved the table nearer a plug and if we put the kettle on the table, he could make coffee. He moved the table and now he can reach the taps over the kitchen sink from his wheel chair.'

Enid stopped for breath and I quickly told Gordon I didn't drink tea or coffee.

Enid seemed to ignore my comments and continued with her narration.

'Do you want me to go on?' and, not waiting for an answer, she went on. 'Our bathroom is upstairs so he can't get to it and Sheila and I have had many battles with him because he doesn't like us bathing him on the bed but the last two mornings Sheila's found him down the garden in the old wash house with a bucket of hot water giving himself a wash and now he doesn't use the commode – he's using the old toilet down the garden, it hasn't been used for years. I wonder it still works! I don't know what's come over him, he's almost human again. He's emptied my washing machine for me and put the washing in the dryer, he's loading the dishwasher and he's turning into a lovely fellow!'

I felt rather embarrassed at hearing such personal details but Gordon cut in with, 'Mum, sit down, shut up and drink your coffee. Let me talk, please! Alan, you don't drink tea or coffee? What can I get you?' and looking at Enid he asked, 'Have you Ovaltine or Drinking Chocolate in?'

She had both and I chose Drinking Chocolate and as I was drinking it, I could feel Gordon's eyes on me and I thought I had to drink this in my own way and show confidence to show him my individuality. After we had finished our drinks, Gordon took Enid by the hand and said:

'Mum, you have done all the talking and Sheila will soon be here and I'd like to talk to Alan. You can stay if you want but please can you not talk?'

Enid smiled, nodded and left the kitchen.

'Right, Gordon, there is a big difference in you. What's happened?'

'You made me think. It's what you said, it's the way you are, maybe it's what you do! You made me realise I have only one life and I've got to live it. No one can help me; I've got to help myself. I want to get things right in my head. I need to accept what's happened to me and get on with it. I don't want to be Mr Nasty anymore. I want to be happy and I want a life. I watched you drink your chocolate this morning and it looked difficult but you don't care, do you? Both Enid and I were watching you and you weren't embarrassed and you just got on with it and you don't care, do you? I want to be like that. Do you know how much I've changed in a few days? These last few days, I've had long conversations with Sheila like we haven't had for two years or more. We have sat at this table and talked to each other and last night we even held hands. I haven't done your homework because I realise what you were trying to do and I'm not dead yet. It's going to be hard work but I'll get there!'

'Where will you get, Gordon? Where is there?'

'Oh Alan, I don't know where there is. But I do know I've got to get my head right. I've got to get my thinking right. I want to talk to you but there's not much time. Sheila will be here shortly.'

'Do you have any money, Gordon?'

'Money, what do I want money for?'

'Because I saw a shop just down the road - why don't you and I go and get Sheila some flowers before she comes home?'

'I can't do that. I haven't been out of this house for ages. What if I meet someone I know?'

'So what, I might meet someone I know. Think about it just a minute. What will your wife's face be like if you give her flowers when she walks through the door and you say I've been out and got these for you? How will you feel now I've offered to push you there and you've imagined your wife's face and you don't go!?'

He was thinking and suddenly he shouted very loudly, 'Mum, can you come here a minute?'

Enid rushed into the kitchen in a panic exclaiming as she rushed through the middle room, 'I'm here, what's up, what's up?'

'There's nothing up, mum. I just want to borrow some money. I'm going down to the shops with Alan!'

Enid looked absolutely flabbergasted; she could hardly speak!

'You're going to the shops. What's got into you?'

'Mum, come on; lend me some money, please. I want to get back before Sheila gets home.'

'Look, my purse is there on the side. Take it with you. I don't believe this!'

Gordon transferred from the dining chair into his wheelchair quite easily. We had to go out from the back of the house and round the side to get to the main road and it took ten minutes for me to push him to the shops. As we approached my car, he asked if I would stop. He wanted to see my car.

'Gordon, it's just an ordinary car!'

Gordon looked wistfully at the car and asked, 'Do you think I'll ever drive again?' 'We'll see! You're not ready yet. We'll see when the time comes.'

'What. You think there's hope?'

'Gordon, there's always hope but leave it for now. Let's go and get the flowers!'

When we arrived at the shops Gordon admitted to feeling excited and I understood. He bought two bunches of flowers, one for Sheila and one for Enid. To buy flowers for Enid was his own idea and I thought it was good.

After paying for the flowers, he was in his chair on the pavement and he asked, 'Do you think you could get me into that shop?' indicating a newsagent's.

'I can have a good try.' And I did. I was surprised as Gordon asked for two boxes of chocolates – one for Sheila, one for Enid.

It was a privilege for me to be there when he gave the flowers and chocolates to Enid. She was overwhelmed and dumbstruck. She did not know what to say! She ruffled his hair, fighting back tears, and in a very croaky voice said:

'Thank you!'

She put the flowers in a vase and scurried into the front room. It was nearly time for Sheila to arrive home and I thought she and Gordon should have a private moment together. I went into the front room to Enid and explained my reasons for leaving Gordon alone.

'Private moment - If he tells her he's been to the shops and bought flowers the shock will kill her! These last three years he has been such a nasty, horrible man. Then you turn up and almost overnight he changes. I tell you, when he called me into that room (pointing towards the back room) after you'd gone the last time and apologised for being selfish and a tyrant, you could have knocked me over with a feather.'

She stopped talking and dabbed at her eyes with a tissue.

'I'll tell you what, we have had some people in this house trying to sort him out but he's seen them off in quick time and when you arrived I thought you'd last two minutes with him. Sylvia, that's his mum, she phoned me and said you were coming and told me all about you and I thought then it's like a lamb to the slaughter. I could not believe you were in with him all those hours. You've had a big effect on him, you know. For the past four days it's been Alan this and Alan that. He's been looking forward to seeing you again. Do you know you are our Sheila's hero!? I don't know what she'll do when she meets you. She may well bow down at your feet!'

I was rather embarrassed at all this praise and quickly hid my feelings in retort.

'Hey, steady on. You'll have me big-headed. I did nothing. He's done the changing, not me. You need to give him the credit, not me. All I did was ask questions and allowed him to talk. He talked a lot more than I. I admit I made him think but I didn't suggest any changes. I did say I wouldn't come back if he didn't clean himself and the room up and I did tell him he and the room stank, but that's about all.'

'Well, whatever you did or said, it worked!'

'Enid, I assure you it's not me. He must have been ready and for some reason I was the right person at the right time and I am so grateful I could be here for him. You know, Enid, my dad used to sing a song. I can't remember all the words but some of them were: if I can help somebody as I pass along then my living will not be in vain – that's my philosophy in life.'

I was aware of voices from the kitchen and I assumed Sheila had arrived home. I'm not very confident in meeting new people and I felt a bit anxious waiting for Sheila to walk in the room. She had obviously entered the house through the back door, which opened into the kitchen. As I stood in the front room, I quickly checked that my tie was straight and that my hair looked okay in the mirror, which hung over the fire place, in anticipation of meeting Sheila.

It was obvious that Enid was a little agitated too as she exclaimed:

'That's our Sheila. I don't know what's keeping her. Should I go and see?'

'No, Enid. Let's leave them she'll come through when she's ready.' And with humour and twinkling eyes, I added, 'Flowers are powerful things and chocolates have even more power!'

Enid's face registered a little smile and we sat in silence for a few minutes, waiting for Sheila.

Sheila eventually entered the room and just threw her arms around my neck and would not let go. Usually when someone hugs me, I put my arms around them and hug them back but I'd never met Sheila before and I am reserved, shy and rather conventional and I didn't know where to put my hands.

Eventually Sheila released me and said, 'I'm so glad to meet you. Alan, you don't know what you've done for my husband.'

Again, I felt rather embarrassed and Enid came to my rescue.

'It's no use talking to him. He won't take any credit. He says Gordon has changed himself.'

'Oh, Alan! Mum and I know different. You have made such an impression on him.'

I shrugged my shoulders.

Sheila turned from me and addressed Enid, declaring,

'I think I got the biggest shock of my life when I walked in the kitchen today. He was sat there with a bouquet of flowers on his lap and he said "I went shopping and bought these for you." Mum, I didn't believe him. Then he produced a box of chocolates. I'm finding it really difficult to believe. Mum, did he really go shopping or did you get them for him?'

'Sheila, Sheila, He did go shopping. I saw him. Alan pushed him and look behind you. I got flowers and chocolates too. I could have fallen through the floor when he came back and gave me flowers and chocolates.'

Sheila's amazement was obvious and she found it difficult to get her head around the flowers.

'Alan, was it your idea to get Gordon to buy me flowers and chocolates? It's incredible. We can't get him to leave the house and suddenly he goes out and buys me flowers. It was all your doing, wasn't it?'

I didn't want to tell any lies or spoil the excitement and surprise so I said,

'I'm guilty of pushing Gordon in his wheelchair to the shops. That's all I'm guilty of.'

Words of astonishment and surprise passed between Enid and Sheila and Gordon's voice interrupted from the kitchen.

'Hey, you lot in there. Have you forgotten me? I'm making sandwiches – come and get them!'

Enid and Sheila looked at each other in complete surprise and one said to the other, 'He's making sandwiches! What next?'

As we all trooped into the kitchen, Gordon indicated that I should sit by him, and as I was sitting down, he thumped my upper arm twice in a very familiar way and looked at me as though we had a secret to share, as though we were in conspiracy together. And I didn't understand what he was trying to convey to me by this gesture.

After we had finished our sandwiches, I uttered that time was getting on and I needed to get home. Gordon was not happy because he wanted to talk to me, so I volunteered to stay for about another hour and he very rapidly moved into the middle room.

I sensed a little awkwardness in Gordon and thought he needed a little help to begin talking so I started the ball rolling by asking:

'You look good but how are you feeling?'

'I'm feeling better and I'm feeling frustrated and guilty. I've realised how I've been with Sheila and Enid in the past and I can't believe I was so nasty.'

He sat for a moment, contemplating and working out what to say next.

'Alan, these last few days have been hell. I've tried so hard to be nice and friendly and helpful. But I can't mooch around the house for the rest of my days doing domestic chores. Surely there's more to life than that?'

'Gordon. You are going too fast. You have made a big change in a short few days. Be proud of what you've done and build on it, but take your time. Don't be impatient! For the past few years all your thoughts, in fact, your whole life, have been taken up by the tragedy of your accident. Your main concern has been how things have affected you. I don't know how I would cope in your situation. The tragedies that have affected your life have rebounded on all your family and I think you're just beginning to see that.'

He was eager to speak. I could see it in his face.

'You are so right, Alan. How can I put all that behind me? How do I build a new life? How do I live with me when I don't like who I am? I really don't want to be like this.'

'Gordon, I'm out of my depth. I can't answer all those questions. Maybe you should look at the alternatives in answer to your questions. Don't think I'm like this all the time – confident… happy… jovial! I have my moments. Negative things happen to me, usually because of an apology for another human being reacting to my disability and, I repeat, I have my moments. But Gordon, I also have a set of core values and a few rules to live by and they help me through.'

'There you go again, Alan, every time you open your mouth you make me think. How do you cope? What are these values and rules?'

'How do I cope? Well, I have my religion and that helps enormously. I have my car – my car is a big asset. It's there I go when I'm upset and frustrated. I put a tape in the cassette player and turn the volume up and I sing as loud as I can and it really helps. I think singing helps my breathing. I do have trouble, my breathing tends to be a bit shallow and singing makes me breath deeper and expand my lungs and that seems to help enormously. But on the other hand, I have a happy home and a wonderfully happy marriage and I refuse to allow my negative feelings to affect my home, especially when those negative feelings are caused by others. What I have at home is really valuable and I'm not too sure too many people have what I have so I treasure it and protect it. I also have a motto, I think you'd call it a motto, it is, "I'll show the buggers!"

I never compare myself to others. I know who I am, I know what I am. I have my life – I live it my way and I love it. I go home at night and lock the door and draw the curtains and I love to be alone with my wife and its absolute bliss! I live for my wife and family.'

113

Gordon was sitting gazing at me and I thought I had talked too much, but he spoke softly and deliberately:

'I do envy you! Do you know what happened this afternoon? I gave Sheila the flowers I bought her, and the chocolates, and she jumped on me, she sat on my knee and she kissed and hugged me and it was terrific. We haven't been that close physically since my accident and hearing you talk about your wife made me decide I'm going to work like hell to get back what we had before we married!'

'That's good, Gordon.'

'It was a good idea of yours to buy flowers for Sheila.'

I hushed him and whispered 'Hey, keep your voice down. She thinks it was your idea.'

'What? And you didn't give me away!?'

'No, I didn't give you away. I think you owe me, don't you?'

After a short pause, Gordon began to talk and he talked for quite some time. I didn't interrupt but his conversation was much more positive than last time. There seemed to be a natural break in his talking and I was eager to get on my way home but before departing I asked about his parents and he replied:

'I'm not ready to see them yet but I will in the future. Sheila and I have talked about it. I need time.'

There are occasions when it's difficult to bring a conclusion to a visit and I really wanted to be on my way. I terminated my visit by advising Gordon that if he needed help, maybe he could go back to his rehabilitation team at the hospital or call his social worker or physiotherapist. To this, Gordon replied emphatically, 'No thank you, I don't think so!'

I took my leave of Gordon, promising to visit again but not saying when. Gordon promised to phone me and I began my journey home. Thinking of what flowers and chocolates had done for Sheila and of course Gordon, I pulled into a garage and bought flowers and chocolates for Kathleen and I thought of her reaction when I gave them to her.

I arrived home and walked in the house and usually I am greeted with a hug and a kiss but on seeing the flowers Kathleen enquired:

'Where have you got the flowers from?'

Anticipating a romantic moment, I announced:

'I bought them for you, darling.'

Her reply:

'You bought them for me? Why? What have you done? What have you been up to?'

And that took the wind right out of my sail!

As I contemplate the change in Gordon, I consider all the experience I've had in living with cerebral palsy and how that experience has added to the man I am. I really feel that if I had not have had my disability and maybe if Gordon had not heard my impeded speech through the door before he met or saw me he would not have accepted me as he did and maybe I could not have helped him as I did. It was such a good feeling to know that I had been instrumental in helping Gordon, Adam and June.

Maybe, just maybe, my disability qualifies me for more than I think!

As promised, Gordon kept in touch with me by telephone. These calls were quite lengthy and usually late in the evening. On one occasion, Gordon spoke about the outhouses at the back of Enid's house and whether they could be converted into a bedroom and en suite bathroom for him and Sheila. I told him to phone his social worker and I further encouraged him by telling him that I had known other people do similar things on a council grant. Two days later, he called me back with great excitement in his voice.

'I talked to my social worker about the extension I'd like and guess what? We are having plans drawn up and the plans and the proposal will go before a committee at the council next month and we may get everything paid for!'

I suppose it was about seven weeks later when I next visited Gordon. He had changed. He was more animated and seemed to be more interested in life. I chose a good day to visit because he had received a letter from the council that morning to say the work on the extension had been approved and a grant was available depending on a social service assessment. I didn't know what it meant and I was surprised at the confidence displayed by Gordon as he rang his local social services, asked them about the assessment and booked an appointment for someone to visit him.

His eyes were gleaming as he returned to me and said:

'That's good, isn't it? Will you come and give me your opinion on what I'd like to do out the back?'

We looked at the proposed project and I encouraged, approved and showed how impressed I was.

We returned in doors and I asked, 'Gordon, what about your mum? Have

115

you contacted her yet?'

Gordon gave a big sigh and answered, 'No, Alan, I haven't. I knew you'd ask but I can't do it and I don't really know why.'

I didn't want to upset him so changed the subject and, picking up the letter, I said,

'I think we should celebrate this. Why don't I take you out for lunch?'

The look on his face told me he wasn't happy. But I insisted and after using my charm and best persuasive – if not bullying – tactics he agreed he would come out to lunch. We decided to go to a pub down the road from his home rather than use my car and go further a field.

I think it took Gordon a little while to get used to the idea and suddenly he started laughing.

'What's the joke?' said I.

'Well, last time you were here we went shopping and bought flowers and Sheila and mum still go on about it and now I have to tell Enid I'm going out to lunch and I'm just thinking about her reaction. She's going to flip her lid! That's why I'm laughing.'

I caught on to his humour and suggested he asked Enid to join us. This brought a twinkle to his eye and a mischievous look to his face and he shouted:

'Mum, Alan and I are going out to lunch. Do you want to come with us?'

Enid arrived in the kitchen immediately, well, in double quick time, looking completely bewildered.

'You're going out to lunch. You're going out to lunch? What do you mean you're going out to lunch?'

'What do you think I mean?'

'Alan and I are going to the pub down the road for lunch. Would you like to come with us?'

Enid's face was a picture and I could see Gordon was enjoying Enid's surprise.

'You are actually going out to lunch and you want me to come with you? I don't believe this. You never leave the house. I'll have to come with you; otherwise I won't believe it.'

I could tell Enid was really baffled and didn't fully believe what was happening and looking at me questionably, she asked.

'Is he for real? I never know, these days. He's wicked. He used to be a grumpy lump but now he teases me all the time!'

'He's for real. Are you coming?'

'I need a minute to get ready.'

'That's okay. We're not in any hurry.'

Enid went off to get ready and Gordon said that he and Sheila had made plans for the future and he had hoped he could run these by me. As he was talking, I thought I could hear voices from the front of the house but Gordon said I was hearing things.

Enid appeared; obviously she had combed her hair and applied makeup.

'I'm ready,' she said, opening the back door, 'Are you pushing him or am I?'

Before I could reply, Gordon said, 'Alan will push me. I don't want you pushing me! You might be temped to push me under a bus!'

Enid ignored this remark and caught us up as we walked down the road after locking the back door.

When we arrived at the pub, Gordon expressed surprise because the door was wide enough for his wheelchair and there was just one small step, which was easy to manoeuvre.

Enid seemed to rush ahead and by the time we got into the restaurant she had already got us a table. As I don't drink, I was ready to order my food but Enid seemed to want to delay.

She ordered drinks from the bar and said, 'Let's take our time and enjoy our drinks; we can eat later?'

I don't know whether it was her manner or her tone of voice which led me to believe she was up to something. We made light conversation until suddenly, Enid said, looking at Gordon:

'Right, me lad. You're not the only one who can pull a surprise!'

No sooner had the remark left her lips than Sheila appeared at our table. Gordon seemed shocked by her appearance and Sheila explained that Enid had called her at work and she had taken an extended lunch break to be with us. We ordered our food and I was really pleased to see the obvious affection between Gordon and Sheila. I was out of my comfort zone. I enjoy having a meal out but I really have to concentrate on the physical aspects: cutting up my food requires concentration; getting the food from my plate to my mouth without spilling it down my front requires concentration. I take my mouth to my hand rather than my hand to my mouth to shorten the journey and this action causes me to appear different and unusual, so I am aware that many people around me tend to stare and watch me eat. This doesn't bother me that much as I always think, 'I'm good enough to be stared at.'

One aspect of my eating does bother me though, and that is my acute gagging reflex. It takes concentrated effort to chew and swallow without gagging, coughing and spluttering. I also need the table and chair to be at the correct height, for this can affect my posture and if my posture isn't correct it affects my hand function and my ability to chew and swallow, etc. So I'm not very talkative whilst at any meal table. I am aware of Sheila saying to Gordon, 'Have you asked him yet?' and Gordon's reply, 'Leave it, I haven't had a chance to talk to him yet and anyway, I'm not sure it's a good idea.'

I assumed the 'him' meant me, so with a questioning look on my face I asked, 'Gordon, Do you want to talk to me about something?'

'No, not really!'

Sheila put down her knife and fork and, touching Gordon's hand and looking searchingly into his eyes, she addressed me:

'Alan, Gordon and I have been talking and he wonders about driving and he wonders about employments. He needs a purpose in life. Can you help him?'

I exchanged glances with Gordon who precipitated my response by hurriedly interjecting, 'It's a stupid idea. It's Sheila, she thinks I could drive. She's so ambitious for me. She wants me to walk before I can crawl.'

I put down my knife and fork, pushed my meal aside and, placing my forearms on the table, I looked Gordon in the eyes and asked, 'Do you want to drive?' to which he replied, 'Yes, I'd like to drive! But that's unrealistic, isn't it? I'm stuck in this thing. I've got to accept things as they are and I don't see myself driving.'

His comments angered me a little and I responded rather aggressively.

'Gordon. You are thinking all wrong. You sound as though your life is over. It's not. If you change the way you think, you will change the way you are. Stop being so negative and pessimistic! Let's find out if you can drive. Ever heard of hand controls? You have got to find out what's available for you. You've got to look at doing things in your own way. I think you can do so many of the things you want to do in life despite being a wheelchair user. You have wonderful support here: Sheila, Enid. Before I leave you today, I'll give you a number to ring to arrange for a driving assessment and after that assessment they will tell you there and then whether you can drive or not. They will also recommend what kind of adaptations you might need and tell you where to get funding if you can't afford the adaptations.'

Gordon's face showed some aggression as he said, 'I can't do that. I don't want to be a charity case! I want to be like other people!'

I could see a sadness creeping over his face and I quickly caught his mood.

'Now come on, I thought we'd got past this. I know it's hard but now you are unique. You are different to others. Just like me. We have to learn to do things our own way and do the best we can.'

I could feel Gordon's anxiety as he retorted:

'I want to be able to pay for what I need. I don't want charity.'

'Oh, piffle, Gordon. I don't want you to be a charity case I want you to find out if you can drive. Can you afford to pay for the car you need? I doubt it! So take advantage of what's on offer and may be in the future you'll be able to pay it back. I'll tell you what, I won't leave that number. You can ring while I'm here and make an appointment and if I can I'll be here to take you for your assessment!'

I sensed that Sheila and Enid were feeling a bit uncomfortable at the exchange between Gordon and me and so I apologised. Sheila said she had enjoyed the performance and couldn't wait to see Gordon behind the wheel of a car.

'I know he can do it!' she said.

She took Gordon's hand, squeezed it and, looking into his face, she said.

'There are times when he feels sorry for himself.'

I came to Gordon's defence and commented:

'Of course there are. But he is doing so well. He is a different man to the one I met a few weeks ago. I don't want to sound patronising but I am proud of him.'

My comment caused Enid to affectionately tease Gordon and I was so glad because that teasing brought relief to the conversation.

After a little while, Sheila asked me if I thought Gordon would ever work. My reply was that I knew many people who used wheelchairs who worked.

Looking at Gordon, I asked, 'What have you done in the past?'

'Well, after university I got a job in the forensic laboratory. I had a really good job with excellent prospects.'

'Sounds good - What did you do at university?'

'I have a degree in the science of applied chemistry.'

As soon as I heard those words, I felt chills running throughout my body because I thought of the vacancy at the pharmaceutical company with the odd bod! My silence was met with stares and questioning looks.

'Something wrong?' asked Gordon.

I shook my head, not knowing how to respond. I didn't want to raise false hopes. Eventually I looked at Enid and said, 'Have you finished your meal? I'd like to go back and use your phone!'

They, all three, looked at me in wonder and I had to say, 'Look, I don't know what to do. I might know of a job opportunity. But I don't want to raise false hopes. Let me make a phone call first and then maybe we can talk.'

Sheila was the one to leave the table first, exclaiming as she did so:

'I'm not going back to work now. This is so exciting. I'll ring and tell them I won't be in this afternoon!'

I did notice that Gordon was rather quiet!

I phoned the odd bod and upon hearing my voice, he said, 'Alan, I knew you wouldn't let me down. You've found someone for this vacancy, haven't you?'

I explained all I could about Gordon. I mentioned his university degree and I did say I wasn't sure if Gordon was the right man for the job.

'We will never know unless we meet him. Bring him along. When are you next free?' Before I knew what was happening, an appointment had been arranged for the following week.

I entered the kitchen where everyone was waiting for news and spoke directly to Gordon.

'I'm sorry; I think I got carried away back there on the phone. I've booked an appointment for you to meet someone to talk with about a job.'

Gordon looked absolutely bewildered and his face registered fear. I could tell that he didn't know what to say and I was beginning to feel guilty and wondered if I had been too pushy.

It was Sheila who broke the stunned silence by saying, 'Tell us more. What kind of a job is it? Where is it?'

I told all that I knew. Sheila's countenance shone with excitement and she and Enid danced around the kitchen but Gordon was subdued! I intervened in the merriment and I had to raise my voice to be heard.

'Look, you two!' I said. 'He hasn't got the job yet. He is going to meet the managing director to talk about possibilities. Don't get carried away. I'd like to hear what Gordon says anyway; he hasn't said a word yet.'

'What do you think, Gordon?'

He looked at me with a doleful, lost puppy look and in a rather quiet voice said, 'I'm scared! I'd like a job somewhere down the line but you're talking about a senior management job. I don't think I could do that?'

I interrupted him.

'Gordon, before you go any further and start putting yourself down, let me tell you, I have a hunch you could do this job and I have a hunch you are going to get on really well with the managing director. I think I know what you're thinking and I've been there and done that. You are not a pathetic disabled person who can't do anything for yourself. You have skills and qualifications, you have abilities and you have talent. Gordon, change the way you think and you will change the way you are!'

Gordon appeared angry at my comments and challenged:

'You make it sound so easy but you can say what you want. I'm stuck in this wheelchair and I'm not the man I was and no matter what or how I think can change the facts!'

'Sorry Gordon, I disagree. I personally have to think positively about myself all the time. I do not ever deny what I am or who I am, but if I listen to others and internalise the negatives, that's how I will act: negatively!'

'Alan, there is nothing negative about you. You're always so positive!'

At this, Sheila came into the conversation:

'Gordon, listen to me please! You have come a long way in a short time! But tell me, when did you last say anything good or positive about yourself? Now look, you have got a really good opportunity here. Go and meet this man. Think how you might do this job. All I've heard so far is "I'm scared. I can't do it". You can do it, I bet you!'

A great deal of encouragement was needed before Gordon said he would go and meet the odd bod and then I wondered if he had said he would go to shut us all up. I thought his acceptance was half-hearted anyway!

The day of the meeting arrived and fortunately I arrived early to take Gordon to his meeting. He wasn't ready! He was having panic attacks and

Sheila, who had taken a day off work, was trying to calm him.

'Gordon!' I said, trying to put authority into my voice, 'What's up? What's the worst that can happen?'

He made no response!

'Gordon. I want to help. Tell me how I can help!'

Still no response!

'Tell me, Gordon, how will you feel tomorrow and in the future if you don't go to this meeting today? Today can affect the rest of your life. Don't let opportunity pass you by.'

At last I had a response, spoken into his beard as it was, 'I suppose you're right. I better go, hadn't I?'

We all breathed a sigh of relief. Enid picked up a shirt from the corner of the room and said, 'I'd better go and iron this again!' and turning to me continued, 'I've ironed it once this morning but he threw it in the corner. It will be crumpled.'

As Gordon was getting ready, I went to my car, phoned the odd bod on my mobile phone and explained the situation. No problems there; he would be available whenever we got there.

Gordon looked amazing in his suit and I had to comment, 'You look like a tailor's dummy.'

He replied bitterly, 'You don't get tailor's dummies in wheel chairs, do you?'

As I was helping him into the car, he said, 'I'm sorry, I can't do this. Please put me back in my wheelchair.' I felt his fear.

'Come on, now. I think I know how you're feeling. Take deep breaths and repeat in your mind, "I can do this, I can do this!"'

'Alan, do you think Sheila could come with us?'

Sheila and Enid jumped in the back seat and off we went.

As we drove along, I wanted to prepare Gordon for his meeting and I tried to start a discussion.

'Hey, you will be positive in the meeting, won't you?'

Gordon looked at me and asked, 'Will you come in with me? I'm really nervous!'

'Hey, I'll support you all I can! Gordon, think of someone learning to parachute. How do you think he might feel before his first jump?'

Gordon again looked at me thoughtfully, 'Really scared, I think.'

'How do you think they might feel when they have become good at parachuting?'

'I get the message, Alan.'

'Not yet you haven't, Gordon! Were you ever scared or nervous before you used a wheel chair?'

'Yes, many times!'

'So, is what you're feeling now to do with your disability or to do with being a normal human being?'

My question went unanswered.

'Can you remember how you felt before your final exam in university?'

Gordon did not respond but I could see he was thinking.

'Gordon. In my life, everything I've achieved has begun with fear. Before college exams, at job interviews, before my wedding, I was scared. Always in my life the excitement and the achievements have begun with fear. Fear has nothing to do with my disability; it's a normal human emotion!'

I could see he was thinking and beginning to smile.

'Alan,' he said, 'You're right! You make me feel really stupid. I can do this, can't I?' I didn't need to reply because there was a chorus from the back seat.

'We've been telling you that all morning!'

We arrived in the car park and as I was helping him into his wheelchair Gordon asked, 'Any more advice?'

'Yes, Gordon. Think what a senior manager might look like. You've got the suit, now think about your facial expression! You've got to look confident and determined!'

'How do I do that?'

'Gordon, what you think in your mind shows on your face. Think and say to yourself, "I am a confident and determined man". Think it and say it from now until the end of the meeting!'

The odd bod greeted us in reception and I was impressed by the way Gordon greeted him. We chatted for a while and were then invited to the odd bod's office and I excused myself. I was asked by Mr Odd Bod to stay close as I might be needed. Twenty-five minutes later, I was called into the office and told that Gordon had got the job if he wanted it but there were a few problems to sort out before Gordon could start. Every problem that came up, I had a solution for and within ten minutes the odd bod was on the phone to the Job Centre, arranging for the Access to Work people to do a workplace assessment. Gordon was then introduced to the man whose job he would be taking over and he was with him for over an hour. Gordon was beaming with delight as he rejoined me in reception, and he asked:

'Can I give you a hug?'

We met Sheila and Enid by my car and before either could say a word, Gordon exploded, 'I GOT THE JOB!'

The relief showing on the women's faces quickly turned to excitement and they hugged each other and jumped and danced around the car park.

Gordon reacted to this joviality by shouting, 'Please, girls, you're the wife and mother of a senior manager. Show a little decorum!'

The assessment that Gordon had for driving proved very positive and before long he became the proud owner of a car and of an electric wheelchair!

It was the middle of October when Gordon started work and almost each day he would call me or leave a message on my answer phone. These calls always started with 'Guess what?' Doors had been widened at work to accommodate his wheelchair, he had interviewed and chosen his own secretary, he and Sheila had been out to dinner with the managing director and his wife and amongst other things, the company had paid the loan off on his car and Access to Work had financed other adaptations and equipment relevant to his needs.

Gordon had also visited his parents and all in all was doing very well.

It was well into the New Year when I received a phone call from Sheila, although I didn't know who the woman was to begin with. As I picked up the phone, a very excited and emotional female voice answered and said all in one breath:

'What have you done to my husband? Do you know what he did? My mum was in on it too, and never said a word to me. He came home from work at lunchtime the day before Christmas Eve and he told me to grab my handbag and get in his car. He said he wanted me to go with him for my Christmas present. I fastened my seatbelt and he said "Your present is in Devon!" He had booked us in a hotel for two weeks. I hadn't packed a thing. He said he had but we were shopping on the way for new clothes and everything else I needed. We've had a wonderful time. Can you believe Gordon could do something like that?'

Had she not mentioned Gordon, I might not have known who it was – so excited was she.

'Yes I can, Sheila. He is doing well! Tell him from me, though, he's in big trouble if my wife finds out about this. She'll expect the same from me!'

I saw Gordon fleetingly on the occasions I facilitated training for the company but there was never time for in-depth discussion on any topic, for I was too involved with my work on those days.

I didn't hear from Gordon for quite a while but I knew he would contact me if he needed me and sure enough, out of the blue, I had a phone call inviting me to lunch with him because he wanted to talk. I had to remind him and explain again, as I have to others, that it's really difficult for me to have a conversation whilst I am having a meal. It takes a great deal of concentration on my part to cut up my food and get it into my mouth without making a mess. So we would eat first and talk afterwards. On my next day off I travelled to his office and arrived a little before the appointed time. He was keen to show me his domain and all the gadgets he had to help him in the workplace. He was a very different man to the man I first met. He had confidence, authority and energy. His electric wheelchair gave him mobility and access. His chair would allow him to change his height so he could reach into cupboards or raise him up to the eye level of others who might stand and talk to him.

He was keen to drive me to the restaurant of his choice and I made approving and appropriate comments about his driving and his car.

After our meal, I wanted to hear what he wanted to talk about but he seemed embarrassed and reluctant and I didn't want to play at twenty questions to find the topic of interest. The only words I could get from him were:

'It's alright for you!'

Eventually, I became rather stern and challenged, 'You brought me all this way just to tell me it's alright for me? Gordon, we haven't time to waste. You need to get back to work and I need to get back home!'

I think he sensed, if not felt, my irritability and responded to my sternness and said, whilst looking around him:

'I'm sorry. It's a bit public here. Can we go and sit in the car and talk?'

I was so impressed by his car! As he opened the driver's door, he positioned himself in front of the gap, pressed a button on his key fob and this fork lift-type thing extended from the car, under the seat of his wheelchair and lifted him; as the wheels of the chair left the ground they folded under his chair and he was placed in his chair in the driving position. Everything in the car was designed to his individual needs. Everything was hand-controlled and convenient to his reach and sitting position. To me it was like magic! When we were both seated in the car, again there was embarrassed silence and I broke it by asking:

'What's bothering you? I can't help if you don't tell me. Talk to me, please!'

He looked at me, nay, stared at me, for a few moments and timidly asked, 'Can I talk about anything to you?'

Frustrated, I replied, 'Gordon, you know you can. Just talk!'

He fidgeted a little and exclaimed:

'I'm embarrassed, but here goes. You know Sheila and I can't do it. We don't have a sexual relationship anymore and I wondered if there was any way we might have children – you know – have sperm taken from me and implanted into Sheila?'

I had learned long ago not to show any kind of emotion and so with a pan face I replied.

'Did the hospital not speak to you about this or at least give you information before they allowed you home?'

'I'm sure they did but I was so frightened and really uncooperative at that time in my life – I really thought my life was over and I didn't take much in!'

I could feel how tense he was, waiting for my reply and I needed to think so I didn't instantly reply; eventually I sorted out my thinking. I had a plan and said:

'Right, Gordon, I've got a plan! Would you speak to someone I know about this? I think you can have sex with Sheila and make your own babies. I just need to make one or two phone calls and set things up for you. What do you think? Will you speak to someone?'

An incredulous and wide-eyed look appeared on his face and with awe and wonder in his voice, he reacted to my question:

'You think I can make my own babies? You're serious, aren't you? You know I'm paralysed down there, don't you? I can't...'

His words faded away and I placed my hand on his forearm and gently and sensitively finished his sentence:

'You can't get an erection! Gordon, I know all that. Would you meet and talk to someone I know who I think might be able to help?'

At the time I was tutoring a group of nurses who were taking a master's course at Luton University; the module I was responsible for involved studies around disability and two of my students were spinal injury specialists. I phoned them, explained Gordon's situation and arranged a meeting.

Gordon rang me after the meeting with one of the students and all he said was that the meeting had gone well and he was excited and needed to speak with Sheila.

About four months later, he rang again to tell me he thought Sheila was pregnant. On enquiring when the baby was due, he said, 'Don't ask me! She's only missed one period but she's always on time, very regular. She must be pregnant!'

It turned out to be true and the baby was born eight months after Gordon's original phone call. Throughout the pregnancy, Gordon phoned me consistently and I had a blow-by-blow account as the pregnancy progressed. Gordon was so excited throughout the pregnancy and he was the proudest of fathers when his daughter was born.

I never discussed how his daughter was conceived. That's private and personal to Gordon and Sheila. But I am intrigued! To be nosey and curious is a sign of intelligent interest and maybe shows how human I am!

CHAPTER SEVEN

I am always amazed at how well I've done in life. I consider myself brainwashed by all the negatives that society threw at me throughout my early years. I had conflict too, for authority and professional people gave me a message of can't do, won't do, while my family encouraged me to do and to try. Both my immediate family and my extended family gave me hope and strength. I remember one meal time when all the family were gathered around the table. It was just before my sister's wedding. There was an argument between Olive, my sister and John, my oldest brother. They were arguing about which of them I would live with and who would look after me on the demise of my parents! John said I would live with him and Olive argued that she would have me live with her. Father intervened and with authority declared:

'Now look, you two, you've been listening to people outside our family! Alan won't need any one of you to care for him when he is older. He is really going to surprise you. Stop arguing and stop saying negative things about Alan. I'm telling you now; he will show you a thing or two when he gets older!' Throughout my younger years my parents, dad in particular, would always combat negative messages with something positive and fortunately I believed my parents rather than those who tried to destroy me. I would suggest that my parents programmed me to think positively. They never denied my disability and they would not allow me to be anything but realistic. They wanted me to be happy with the person I was and they wanted me to be in control rather than allow others to control me. It was as though my father had been primed before my birth for he always knew what was best for me and always made me feel of value. He had realistic expectations for me and he led my mother and the family in caring for me.

I was twenty-seven when I first met Kathleen. I lived on my own at the time. I rented a one bedroom flat and I had a really good life. I had many female friends and had had numerous 'girlfriends'. Never had marriage ever entered my head. I didn't want to be married and didn't ever analyse why this was. It could have been that I didn't want the responsibilities connected with marriage. It could have been that subconsciously I didn't consider myself husband material or maybe I just hadn't met the right person. However, I met Kathleen and she took over my mind. I was absolutely obsessed by her. My waking thoughts were of Kathleen and at the close of my day she was on my mind and I could not understand why. I didn't like what was happening to me; it felt like I was being taken over by another person. The funny thing was I'd never been alone with her. I had talked with her but always in public and, looking back, whenever she had the opportunity she would always seek me out. It took months for me to ask her out on a date. Usually I didn't have any problems in asking a girl to partner me at a dance or to go to a show or whatever with me and if they refused I would not be hurt or offended; I would always move on to the next girl. With Kathleen it was different. Had she to turn me down or shun me, I would have been destroyed and rather than allow that to happen, I kept her at arm's length. I was friendly but that's all! I tried for months to get Kathleen out of my mind. I felt guilty because I could not stop thinking of her. When she said yes to our first date I felt like 'fizz bombs' were fizzing throughout my body. (Fizz Bombs are tiny sweets that fizz on your tongue when you suck them!) Even though it's long ago, I vividly remember our first kiss. Wow. That first kiss! I was captivated. I was floundering like a fish on the end of the line! When Kathleen accepted my proposal of marriage I almost burst with pride and excitement. Even after over forty four years of marriage and rearing three children I still feel the same. She occupies my every thought and I am obsessed with her. My delight is to lock the door to our home, close the curtains, shut out the world and be with Kathleen, just the two of us on our own. It's absolute bliss. In my home I find solace; it is my sanctuary, particularly when I am there alone with Kathleen! My relationship with Kathleen instils in me a lively consciousness of existence, for in that relationship I recognise my ultimate success and the very core of my reason for living.

Always has Kathleen had high expectations of me and has supported me in any ambition I've had. She is always down to earth and direct in any advice she offers. She never criticises but will always discuss. She never puts me down but always builds me up and encourages. She makes me feel like a real man like no one ever has or could.

Kathleen knows me so well and when I fall apart she is always able to put me back together, like the time I took my four-year-old grandson to the local play park. This four year old was my first grandchild! We were having a great time. I'd push him high on the swings and he'd giggle. He enjoyed the roundabout, and most of all he loved the big slide as I caught him at the bottom and tickled him. We were having such a happy time until we were joined by a lad of seven or eight years of age who obstructed all our play! He would sit on the bottom of the slide or climb up the slide the wrong way so that my grandson couldn't slide down or stand in front of the swing so I couldn't push it without hitting him. I asked this young lad to join us. I suggested we play together, to which he replied, 'Don't you talk funny? Talk some more so that I can laugh!' Usually this kind of comment wouldn't bother me but as it was said in front of my grandchild I was perplexed! Kneeling down in front of the offending boy, I started to explain about my speech when a woman approached and angrily asked, 'What are you doing with my son?' I arose from the ground and explained what had happened. The woman gathered her son to her and shouted at me as she walked away, 'Well, you do talk bloody funny and if you don't want to be laughed at you should stay indoors.' I couldn't retaliate as the woman was walking away from me at a great pace and really my concern was for my grandchild. I was somewhat distraught; not really at what had been said, because throughout my life there has always been someone to remind me of my differences in a negative way, but that my grandson had witnessed and heard the incident. As Kathleen and I were discussing what had happened and as she was administering TLC to me and explaining things to our grandchild, our doorbell rang and on answering its call I found three teenage girls on my doorstep who said they had seen and heard the activity on the playground and had come to see if I was alright. I was encouraged by the kindness and concern of these young women. They were also able to tell me who the woman was and where she lived!

I don't consider myself to be very brave but I mustered up sufficient courage to go and knock on the woman's door and gently confront her. I first of all apologised for the shock it must have been to her when she saw me with her son. Then I asked how she thought I felt at the words she flung at me in front of my grandchild. Fortunately, the woman had calmed down and we were able to discuss the situation calmly. Ever after that, whenever I saw the woman or her son, they would wave and say hello and sometimes stop and chat (I must clarify the extent of my bravery as I went to challenge this woman – I did take my dog with me).

Business was booming for me and we were really busy. I hadn't seen

Adam for two or maybe three years. I often thought about him but never had enough time to visit him. I knew if he needed me, he would contact me! Sure enough, a call came early one Saturday evening; Adam spoke excitedly down the phone.

'Alan, we want you to be the first to know June and I are engaged! We got engaged last night and we are getting married. Will you come?'

I replied with enthusiasm, 'That is good news, Adam. When is the wedding?'

'Don't know yet but will you come?'

'Adam, you let me know when the wedding is and if I can, I'll be there!'

The phone went dead. I suppose Adam had got the answer he wanted but was too excited and distracted to make polite conversation or indeed to give any more details.

We did attend the wedding and it was a lovely affair. I was so impressed by both bride and groom. Adam looked so handsome in his new grey lounge suit and June looked absolutely stunning in a white dress with a very full skirt which accentuated her small waist and trim figure. Her dress was trimmed with frothy lace with sparkling diamantes and seed pearls. Her dad looked so proud as June walked down the aisle of the church on his arm. I doubt if the bride's mother's tears exceeded those of the bridegroom's parents. When the bride threw back her veil at the appropriate part of the ceremony her smile was dazzling.

I was led to think how man needs woman because I could see how Adam had developed. He had a certain stature and an assurance as he stood by the side of his bride and June had developed a confidence and maturity. He also appeared confident and he certainly had charisma! As with all weddings I attend, I am made to reflect on and contemplate my own marriage and I know I would not be the person I am without Kathleen in my life. I think having someone to care for and having the responsibility of the support of a family is the ultimate in personal development. It would be so easy for me to indulge in my own problems and it is good for me to have others to care for; others whose welfare and happiness come before my own.

I do find it very thrilling to reflect on my past life. I feel it a great privilege to know and work with people like June and Adam and to be part of their growth and development. I also contemplate that I was the one who brought them together. Isn't life wonderful!? It was at this time I discovered that I had another disability. A rather embarrassing one! 'Incontinence of the eyeballs'!

I had, by this time, developed a reputation as a trainer and I travelled extensively. My work was divided between disability equality awareness training and employment equality training. I was really happy with the feedback I received on my courses and research showed that many companies had changed their policies and practices and many disabled people had been employed through the effect of my training.

A central government department invited me to a meeting to talk about my work, supposedly. But actually the discussion focused on the status and designation of disabled employees in the department. It was found that ninety eight per cent of employees with disabilities were in the bottom, lower-paid band of the organisation. Disabled employees didn't seem to gain promotion! The meeting looked at statistics and each person present had much to say. The meeting went on and I began to wonder why I had been invited to attend because I had not made any contribution and the meeting seemed not to include or offer any questions for me. Eventually the chairman addressed me and explained my presence, 'You were invited here so that you might become aware of our concerns and issue. Your reputation is well-known to this Department and we want you to design a course which will give our people the confidence to apply for promotion and the skills required to achieve it.' It seemed unusual to have this kind of offer from a government department. I had gone through a long and complicated tendering process to gain a contract for other training I did for this and other government departments so it was difficult to believe I was being offered work without having to tender for it. However, it was explained that this work was offered to me as an extension to my existing contract.

Although I was rather chuffed at being offered this extension to my contract, it gave me cause for thought. Initially my immediate thoughts were rather negative.

I wondered what I had to offer to such a training course. It took me a little while to reason things out. After all, I had life experience and I had been trained by experience to cope effectively with my differences, so I concluded my thoughts by affirming to myself that I had lots to offer to such a course. I developed a positive attitude and began asking questions of other disabled people and created a four-day training programme.

My feelings were that if I were to achieve the aims and objectives attached to this contract, the people responsible for promotion in the department needed to be involved in the training, if not needed training themselves.

It took a great deal of research and thought to design a programme for the proposals and in working on this I became aware that the contract I'd been given was restrictive to achieving what had been explained to me at the initial meeting. I presented the proposals for the training programme – along with specific recommendations – to the department's training manager and to my surprise they were accepted! This meant that the content of my contract increased in terms of the number of courses I had to facilitate and in terms of the value of the contract. Whereas initially, four one-day courses per year were offered, we now had four residential courses of four days' duration with line manager involvement in action planning and one-day training courses for line managers. In addition to this, we were to organise a three-day conference each year where delegates were to be invited back to feed back on progress and be 'refreshed' on the aims, objectives and philosophy of the four-day course! The whole project excited me and had grown exceedingly. I was nervous, to say the least, for I hadn't engaged in this type of work before. It was akin to personal development training and I really had little experience in this area.

The aims and objectives of the courses were publicised but my orientation and game plan were important to the success of the course and I wasn't too sure that I had the skill, knowledge or experience to have successful outcomes from this course. These doubts and uncertainties are always good for me, they allow me to be humble and not take things for granted. They make me more conscientious and thorough in my planning and maybe in my presentation as well. Alan the trainer is a very different person to Alan the ordinary man. Ordinarily, I tend to be a little timid and shy but in the training room I have to present an air of confidence and power. Always, I perform a little ritual before I begin a training course. Usually, I sit waiting for the last delegates to arrive or for the appointed time to start and always, I will slap the table in front of me with my hand or slap my thigh if there is no table. That slap causes me to enter the role of a trainer and somehow causes a change to take place within me.

Kathleen and I awaited the date of the first course on this new contract and it came all too soon.

CHAPTER EIGHT

The Department had booked a training venue on the site of a large hotel in central England that had an excellent reputation and a protected and secure environment. Kathleen and I arrived early, long before the course was due to start because we needed to be organised and we needed to find our way around the venue.

At reception, we were greeted by a female receptionist and I gave her my name and introduced my wife. I told her I was the trainer for the course. I was horrified by her reaction: 'You're the trainer!' she said in a surprised manner, 'and this is your wife!' and continued, 'How can you be a trainer?' I was speechless and momentarily stunned, and before I or Kathleen could respond, the receptionist walked off into an office behind reception. I could see into this office from where I was standing in reception and through my experience of working in a cotton mill, I can lip-read! The receptionist was reporting to a man in the office and commented on the way I was dressed – I was dressed casually. I intended to change into my suit later. She commented on my speech and she commented on her assumptions about my intellect and mental capacity. She also told the man, 'He says he is married to that woman!' I was aware that the staff at the hotel had been alerted to security issues in housing the course – we were at risk because we came from a central government department, but I was not at all happy at my reception. The man who the receptionist had spoken to approached me in reception and tried to take me to one side in the reception area, out of public view! 'I'm sorry!' I began, 'I'm not budging from here. What business we have can be done right here on this spot.' I fumbled in my pocket for my wallet and pulled out my driving licence, which had my photograph on it. 'Right now, sir, you know who I am. I am really angry at the welcome I have not received and at the assumptions of that apology for a receptionist.' I really felt the man was trying to blame me as he said, 'The receptionist was only doing her job. We are on a security alert and no one told us you were disabled!' I cannot repeat my reply! I really was furious. Not only had I been insulted but my confidence had been affected. I was offered no apology either. I am very careful on occasions such as this that I do not internalise negatives. I looked at the man questioningly and mentally willed him to offer me an apology but after a brief pause, none was forthcoming. So I suppose I went on the attack and, using a business-like voice, I looked the man in the eye and began, 'My first job is to check the bedroom of every student on my list to make sure that all their requirements are taken care of. Can we do that now, please; I assume that the Department has sent you a list?'

'Yes, I have it in my office.'

'Could you get that list please? Wait a minute though. Could my wife – (taking Kathleen gently by the arm)... Sorry, we haven't got our marriage certificate with us but she and I know we are married. Could Mrs Counsell sign in and get the key to our room, please, whilst you and I go through the list, please?' My anger was controlled and gave me strength to command this younger man. I really was furious!

I think the receptionist tried to apologise to Kathleen, for I heard her say, '"Sorry", I think you might be by the end of the week!' and off Kathleen went to our room as the man returned with his list. I assertively took the list from him and placed it on the counter between us, where could both see it.

'We have three wheelchair users. Have you assigned wheelchair accessible rooms?'

'Yes, we have. These are larger than the other rooms.'

'I should hope they are. But are the doorways wider and where is the toilet placed in the bathroom?'

The man looked really puzzled and spoke to me with some annoyance, 'I don't know what you mean. The toilet is in the bathroom, that's all I know.'

'I'm sorry, that's not good enough. I don't know how these people transfer from their wheelchair to the toilet so we really need to be able to get a wheelchair at each side of the toilet. Each wheelchair user is different. Some may need to transfer to the right, some to the left, whilst others may transfer from the front.'

The man had an incredulous look on his face and confessed, 'I don't know! I've never thought about it before! Can you and I go and look at one of our disabled rooms?'

I could tell I had got this man worried - which was my aim!

'I am sorry but I have much to do to prepare for my students. I really haven't time to look at rooms. Could you get someone to check with the students when they arrive, please? I suggest you have a member of staff escort the wheelchair users to their bedrooms and make sure everything is convenient for them. Now, look, we have a woman on our list with visual impairment. Apart from her needing large print, I don't know what other needs she may have. For example, will she be able to see the number on her bedroom door – can she see the keyhole and insert her key easily? I don't want her trying to get into the wrong room after she's had a drink in the bar, one evening!'

This man was really worried now and said, 'There's a lot more to this than meets the eye. What do I need to do for this woman who is visually impaired?'

'Let's wait and meet her, and Mrs Counsell will work with her if need be. We've brought bits and pieces with us; that may help.'

We continued to go through the needs of my students and I was enjoying myself in pointing out how ill-prepared the hotel was, knowing full well that each student would cope, for they would be used to encountering inconvenience in their lives.

I was getting a little apprehensive about time. I really had a lot to do before the students arrived and I wanted to get on. So I said, 'I'm sorry, I've got to go. I have to unpack my car and organise my training rooms. I've a lot to do. My last concern is your receptionist. I have twenty-two students arriving; all have disability. I really don't want them treated or greeted as I was!'

'Don't worry about that. It will be alright. Honestly, it will.'

I moved closer to the receptionist so that she could hear me and replied:

'You have more confidence in your receptionist than I have. She didn't think I should or could be married. She thought I could not be a trainer and she thought I was mental. You see, I can lip-read so I knew what she said to you back there in the office! I do hope she is not on reception when my people arrive. I'm also very concerned that we have other courses booked at this establishment in the future!'

I left two very red-faced people at reception as I walked away to find Kathleen.

Kathleen had been busy. She had unpacked the car and organised our bedroom and was on her way to organise the training room.

It may have seemed that I had coped well with the rebuff of the receptionist but it had affected me greatly. On the surface, I might have appeared able to cope but underneath, I was somewhat disturbed. I suppose I felt like a swan gliding sedately on the water but paddling like mad underneath. I really wanted to feel good. Students are important to me and I always want to give of my best to them. To do that, I need to feel good and the incident at reception on my arrival had knocked my confidence. I was angry at myself for allowing the incident to get to me so much and I was still furious at the receptionist!

Often I experience such an encounter which reminds me of my disability and the attitudes of others, reinforcing negatives and bringing back memories that I wish I could forget! Why is it so easy for others to destroy me? Why do I have to assert myself? Why can't the positive messages of my family be reinforced and instantly remembered by me rather than the awful traumas and negatives of my childhood?

Of course, as per usual, Kathleen came to my rescue.

'Alan, you've time for a shower and we have time to talk and listen to some music! So get on with it and I'll go and sort the training room out. You relax and let things go. Think positive! You're a really good trainer! Now relax!' With this, she administered a strengthening hug and left the room.

I got myself dressed and looking as smart as I could and Kathleen returned to the room: 'Everything is organised and you look great. Can we go to the car for ten minutes? And then we are going to the restaurant for lunch!'

'But we don't have lunch booked!'

'Ho, ho, ho. We do now. That man you spoke to in reception – he came and had a word with me. I think he's frightened of you he said you were formidable and we have a complimentary lunch waiting for us in the restaurant. I've also arranged for two of the hotel staff to carry students' luggage from their cars when they arrive and, and, I haven't finished yet, there's complimentary refreshments for the students when they arrive - all these goodies because you attacked the receptionist!' (The word 'attack' was said smilingly and with mischief in Kathleen's eyes.)

I was feeling somewhat better and by the time we'd sat in the car, listened to music and had an excellent lunch, my inner confidence was restored.

Because Kathleen had organised everything so well, I had very little to do! My one remaining task was to go through the programme for the afternoon and make sure I knew what I was doing. This didn't take me very long and we decided to go and sit in reception and meet the students as they arrived. I'm glad we did! The reception area was lit with decorative lighting on the wall behind the reception desk. It was not good lighting. Several things happened. One student who had declared that he had a hearing impairment and used lip-reading arrived. I met him by the door and knew who he was because he was wearing his departmental identity. I purposely introduced myself just inside the entrance to the hotel where there was lots of natural light. I strategically placed myself so that the natural light was on my face to make lip-reading easier.

'Hello Tim. I'm Alan and I'm your trainer. Did you have a good journey? Did you drive?'

'No. I came by train and got a taxi from the station. It looks an impressive hotel.'

'Yes, Tim, the hotel is good. We are in an annex in the grounds. Our bedroom is really nice and my wife and I had lunch and the food is excellent!'

'That's good. I like my food.'

'Tim, I am a little concerned. I do have difficulty with my speech and I know you lip-read. Are you okay with me? Can you read my lips okay?'

'Alan, I have no problem understanding what you are saying. You're great. Thank you for asking. You've just put me at ease. I'm really going to enjoy my week.'

Tim went over to reception to register and get his room key! Oh dear, he had great problems at the reception desk. The lighting was behind the receptionist, which is not conducive to lip-reading, and the receptionist kept her head down, looking at her computer screen whilst talking to Tim. I walked over to Tim and took over from him. I addressed the receptionist, a different one to the one I met earlier. 'Have you found Tim on your computer?'

'Yes, I have, but who are you?'

I had been seen from the office and the man I had spoken with earlier in the day hurried from the office.

'Is everything alright there, Mr Counsell?'

'I'm afraid not. This young man relies on lip-reading and the lighting is awful and the receptionist keeps her head down when she is speaking to him. He hasn't a clue what is being said to him. I was going to point out that it tells her on her computer that he lip-reads.'

The man looked at me with a look of frustration on his face! 'I am sorry! You had better come through to the office with me!' It took two minutes to book Tim in because the office was well lit and the man looked at Tim each time he spoke to him.

As I left the office, Kathleen was stood at the reception desk with a woman who I assumed was a student. As I approached, Kathleen called me over: 'Alan, this is Stella.'

'Hello Stella, I'm Alan and I'm your trainer for this week. We'll talk later when you've signed in.'

The receptionist tapped her pen on the counter and asked Stella to sign her name in two places. Stella asked for a template and the receptionist asked, 'I don't know what you mean. What do you want a template for? I just need your signature.'

Stella looked at the receptionist and said, 'I don't see very well. Not in this light anyway, and I need a template to help me to write my name in the right place!'

The receptionist looked from Kathleen to Stella and a broad grin appeared on her face.

'It's a joke, isn't it? You don't look blind. Has my colleague put you up to this?' Stella looked enraged and angrily said, 'I assure you this is no joke. I am not blind as you call it but I do have a visual impairment and I can't see to sign my name. I need a template!'

'I'm sorry? I don't know what you mean. I don't have a template and I'm still not sure this is not a wind up!' she looked incredulously at Kathleen.

Kathleen is usually calm and collected but on this occasion she became rather ruffled and took command of the situation by putting up her hand as though she were stopping traffic and saying to the receptionist, 'Enough, enough! I know the office sent a template. I'm coming round there!'

Kathleen walked around the counter, fumbled about and produced a template. She looked at the receptionist and said, 'This is a template and look on your computer; it says in red – "Stella has visual impairment and requires a signature template". Look, it tells you there!'

Kathleen touched Stella's arm over the counter so that Stella was aware that she was going to speak directly to her.

'Stella, did you hear all that? I've got the template. I'll place it on the paper. Give me your hand.'

Kathleen placed Stella's hand on the template and Stella felt for the space and signed her name. The whole process took a matter of seconds!

A template is a piece of rectangular plastic with a space cut large enough for people like Stella to write their signature. The plastic is thick enough to allow people to feel the cut-out space placed over the appropriate place on the form.

We had a few more incidents at reception. Wheelchair users couldn't reach the high counter and Kathleen produced a clipboard so they could sign in on their lap. Two people who had requested a bathroom with a shower had been given a room with a bath and the receptionist haughtily said, 'There is a shower over the bath!'

So we had to explain that these two people had both got back problems that affected their mobility and they could not get into a bath. Kathleen produced a copy of the documentation that had been sent to the hotel concerning students' needs and these two people had very specifically requested 'a walk-in shower, no bath.'

As the students were enjoying their refreshments, I was approached by a young man who asked if he could speak to me in private. We found a secluded corner and he introduced himself.

'I'm Peter and I have epilepsy! I haven't had a fit for ages, so I'll be okay this week. I just thought you should know but I don't want anyone else to know!'

'Alright Peter, I'll respect your wishes. But! Why don't you want the others to know?'

'For many people there is a stigma attached to epilepsy and people shun me because they are scared I might have a fit in front of them and I want to make friends this week. I haven't had a fit for ages. So I don't need people on the course to know.'

'Peter, I'm not happy. I can cope. I'm not afraid and I won't shun you but if you did have a fit, would the people around you be less affected if they knew?'

'No. I won't have a fit this week. I haven't had one for ages and I don't want people to know!'

I had to respect Peter's wishes but I wasn't happy!

CHAPTER NINE

The training room was light, airy and quite large. All the chairs were of the same design and I knew these would not be comfortable for some of our students. After formal introductions, Kathleen and I did what we call an audit of need. We explained to the students that they were going to sit in this room or in a syndicate room for the next four days and we wanted them to be comfortable. We were also concerned about their bedrooms: were they comfortable, did they need more pillows – whatever they needed, we wanted to know. So they had to tell us what they needed and we would try and get it for them. Kathleen created a list and she went off to reception to talk about extra pillows, non-slip mats for baths and showers and extra towels in individual bedrooms. I went in search of three high-backed chairs for students with back problems, two foot rests, and a swivel chair for Tim so that he could turn around and lip-read people behind or to the side of him in group discussions. Tim also needed a television with subtitles in his bedroom. I think Kathleen spoke with the housekeeper and everything needed for the bedrooms was supplied but we literally had to steal the chairs we needed from various offices. People working at the hotel were reluctant to give up their chairs but, by fair means or foul, I acquired all that was needed.

We had two people with repetitive strain injury and we thought they might have trouble with their bedroom keys so we gave them a key holder, which made the key longer, bigger and much easier to handle. We also stuck brightly-coloured fluorescent paper around the keyhole and around the number on Stella's bedroom door, allowing her to see where to put her key and to recognise her room easily.

We then established a strict code of confidentiality with the group. And we laboured this heavily. We stressed that anything that was said which was of a personal nature must not be repeated outside of the course. We wanted people to have confidence to speak up and say what they wanted, knowing that what they said would not be repeated, belittled or laughed at. We emphasised that everyone's contribution would be valued. I also explained that in my opinion there were no experts in disability! I explained that I considered the experts to be the people who have personal experience and live with it twenty-four hours a day. I am an expert on me and my views and opinions are based on my experiences, so I value the expert opinions of those in the room. We wanted each person to accept, respond and add to our code of confidentiality and Kathleen and I were both surprised when comments were made on how we had made the group feel so welcome and how our concern for their comfort had impressed them. We felt that we had an instant rapport with the group. Before I could begin training, I needed to make sure I knew what needs people had in the training room in order for them to gain the most from the course. I felt that Stella was sitting in the wrong place and asked if she would like to move so that her back was to the window rather than having strong light on her face. Her reaction was rather animated. 'Alan, who the hell are you? Do you have magical powers? I was just thinking I should have sat over there and I hadn't the confidence to say anything!'

Instantly, people moved around and allowed Stella to sit with her back to the window. Mischievously, hoping she would understand my humour, I touched her arm and I said, 'Stella, I have a problem with you. How do I know whether you've gone to sleep or whether you're just resting your eyes?'

'I won't go to sleep, honestly!'

This was a lead-in to my next question to the group.

'I don't want to know about your medical label but I do need to know what you need in the training room to gain the most from this training.'

I allowed the group a little time to think and added:

'For example, Stella will need to rest her eyes from time to time, not because she is sleepy but because of other issues. She also needs people to read out to her what they have written on a chalkboard or flipchart or OHP that's both in the large group or smaller syndicate groups. If we show a video, Stella will need someone sat by her to give a commentary of the activity on the screen. Am I right, Stella?'

'Alan, you're spot on. I don't know how you know all these things!'

'Is there anything else, Stella?'

'No, Alan, you've covered everything!'

'I have talked about need and not your medical label.'

And addressing the group, I ask, 'What's more important, need or diagnosis?'

The whole group discuss this and the consensus of opinion was that need was more important than diagnosis but sometimes people didn't know what they needed.

So again, with devilment in my eyes, I addressed Stella.

'Stella, do you have any other needs?'

'No, I think you've covered them.'

'What about in the dining room? Would it be helpful if people told you what was on your plate and where it was? You know – potato at two o'clock, peas at six o'clock?'

'Yes, that would be helpful. I was hoping to make a friend before dinner to do just that for me!'

Many people in the room volunteered to sit by Stella at dinner and assist her.

'Stella – what about in the bar tonight? Can you pay for your own drinks or would someone else need to pay?'

I realised that Stella could not see my facial expression and might miss the ambiguity of what I was saying.

When the majority of the group laughed, Stella realised the humour in my words and responded:

'You know exactly what I need.'

'Tim, it's your turn next. Tell us what you need in the training room?'

'I don't hear very well and I rely on lip-reading. I need to be able to see people's faces when they're speaking.'

Looking directly at Tim, I responded:

'Is lip-reading tiring? Does it take a lot of concentration? What I'm concerned about is the amount of talking this week, from me, from Kathleen and from the group. Will you cope?'

'Yes, Alan, I am sure I'll cope. I bet you have lots of written hand-outs for me, haven't you? All the videos you'll show will have subtitles too, won't they?'

'You're right, Tim! But if you need time out, let me know. Tell me why you've got a swivel chair?'

'So that I can swivel round and look at people when they're talking behind me! This chair will save my neck!'

'But Tim, how will you know people are talking behind you if you can't hear them?'

'I am hoping people will tap me on the shoulder and show me who's speaking!'

'Is there anything else, Tim?'

'I don't think so. You have made me feel so comfortable. I'm going to enjoy this week.'

'Can you cope if more than one person speaks at the same time?'

'No. I can't cope with that.'

'So, Tim, you need us to speak one at a time?'

'Yes, that's right. I'm useless in a group if everyone speaks at the same time! I'm better in a one to one.'

'Tim, can I ask you a personal question?' I asked, looking directly at him and hoping he could see the humour in my face.

Tim turns around and addresses the group: 'What's coming now? Look at his face, it's full of devilment.' And turning to face me, he said, 'Go on, ask me what you want!'

'Tim, is it true you have a vibrator in your bedroom?' the room went really quiet and the students looked rather shocked as they awaited Tim's response.

'O that! It's true. I do have a vibrator in my bedroom (Tim paused for effect). It's a pillow vibrator. I can't hear an alarm clock so I have a device which vibrates under my pillow and wakes me up at the time I want it to.'

The majority of the group laughed at my ambiguity and some remarked that they had never heard of a pillow vibrator!

After more discussion of individual needs and domestic issues, I felt that Kathleen and I had developed a good relationship and a good rapport with the group.

When the group had arrived, they had been a little tense, particularly those who encountered difficulties at reception. They may have felt tired too: travelling can be stressful and tiring, particularly if one has a visual impairment. Just imagine sitting on a train and there's no announcement from the conductor and you can't see where you are and the people sitting by you constantly come

146

and go. Each time the train stops, you have to ask where you are and everyone tells you there is a digital indicator screen at the end of the carriage. Each time, you have to reply and tell people you're blind. I think I might feel vulnerable and I might be reluctant to travel. Certainly, the tension would tire me!

Kathleen and I had worked hard to put people at their ease and in talking about and supplying individual needs, we hoped we had made them feel important, comfortable and welcomed. I had also injected humour wherever I could because I feel appropriate laughter causes people to feel good and makes them relax.

It was now time to get down to some serious work!

I knew the first exercise would be rather controversial. The delegates had to define 'disability'! It really is not easy to do! In my own life, I carry a mental definition of my identity! Society, in general terms, is usually rather negative in defining who I am. People tell me I am a 'disabled' person. I refuse to go along with the thinking behind this label! When those three letters, 'dis', appear before any word, they negate the word which follows, thus 'dis' negates 'ability'. I have lots of ability and so I need to define myself in terms of ability. As predicted, there were lots of negatives in the students' definitions of disability and the ensuing discussion was powerful and controversial! My purpose in beginning the course in this way was to get the students to think. I also wanted students to analyse why they had defined disability so negatively. Had they defined it using their own experience, from what others said about disability, from the current political language or some other input? In fact, I wanted to know if they really believed their own definitions and if they did, how were they affected by their definitions in terms of self value, self confidence and their own internal thoughts? It is so easy to internalise negatives and personally, I need my internal language, my innermost thoughts, to be positive, for who I am and what I am is determined by what I think and I am always on my guard, for I am bombarded by negative messages. I would rather be affected by the rationalised truth, which I carry around within me, than by myths, assumptions and stereotypes that others bandy about with obscene abandon.

Always, this session creates wonderful and diverse discussion. Always too, would I be asked for my definition! And it is: 'Disability is a positive life style which encourages achievement using personal creativity and initiative.' Again, this created interesting discussion but ultimately it made people think and for me, thinking affects the way I function. I consider my mind to be my strongest defence in dealing with the negatives around disability and if I have a positive image of myself, in my inner being, and can define myself in a positive way, I am going to be a formidable opponent in any battle. Many use the word 'impairment' in defining disability and again I have to challenge. To me, the word impairment conjures up comparisons and these comparisons are against a set of norms. If I don't measure up to these norms then I am impaired or weakened. One meaning of the word impaired is weak! I really have to object because the effects of my medical label strengthen me in every way! All this is said to stimulate discussion and to allow thinking to take place. These definitions are my own, they appertain to my life and they actually work for me. I do not expect everyone to accept my thinking; I merely want people to think about their own inner language and their own thoughts and the effect of these on their identity!

Each of us is uniquely individual. I can learn from others and I greatly value the thoughts and philosophies of others.

For a few of those in our group who had recently acquired disability, the discussion was different because the change from identifying oneself as a non-disabled person into identifying oneself as a disabled person can be really traumatic, particularly if one's thinking on disability had been negative before acquiring the identity.

Change is never easy. Life changes all the time for all of us and very often we don't have a choice. Sometimes we create change to better our lives. But to change one's identity is a mammoth change and depending on the acquired disability, it might involve many people: spouse, family and colleagues. It can take an insurmountable length of time to accommodate a newly acquired disability and I am aware of how my definition could affect others who may not be ready to philosophise!

I would suggest, though, that there are some who need to look at their attitudes because very often if one doesn't manage change, change will manage them.

I believe the loss element around acquired disability can be great and very often, it's never talked about! Just one example of this might be the loss of the home one had.

If one becomes a wheelchair user – how does one accommodate a wheelchair into one's home? One may have a modern home with a coordinated colour scheme and matching chairs, etc. To accommodate a wheelchair, one may have to rearrange furniture and may interfere with the design and layout of a home. I suggest that the loss of such things could have a tremendous impact on many family members and it is hardly ever mentioned in conversation or counselling.

I obviously don't have an acquired disability and therefore haven't experienced any of the issues involved but my role as a trainer is to make people think. Very often, knowledge is required to manage an acquired disability. I do not deny the traumatic impact of an accident or disease that causes one to acquire disability but ultimately, a person needs to know what equipment, etc., there is available and from meeting many who have acquired disability, I am aware of a severe lack of knowledge and awareness. This lack inhibits choice and a lack of choice can cause a lack of self-management and I suggest that if we do not manage our needs, our disability will manage us. If we are not in control and if our needs are not met then our definition of disability might be negative, as might our own self-image!

Very often during this defining exercise, people would become somewhat heated as I challenged some of their negative thinking but always, during the refreshment break which followed, many people would come and talk to me and admit they needed to change the way they thought!

Usually, during this short refreshment break, the discussion continues and students interact and bond with each other. I believe that the way I define 'disability' in my own mind is really important because the language other people use to describe me and define me can be so negative and I combat these negatives by being realistically positive and being proud of who I am and what I am. I want the students to have an opportunity to discuss and think about these issues.

The second session is for students to discover what causes their disability! I have met lots of disabled people who actually blame themselves rather than the actual cause of 'inability'. For example, I have difficulty using an ATM; my dexterity is such that I can accidentally punch in the wrong PIN and on numerous occasions, my card has been swallowed up, so I go into the bank and ask a cashier when I want to withdraw money from my account. Often I am told I have to use the ATM; I do get fed up of explaining my predicament and it would be so easy to blame myself! Delegates are asked to discuss my problem with ATMs, discuss some of their own experiences and discover the many causes of disability. It's amazing where this session usually leads! Numerous barriers are recognised. The attitudes in society are realised as possible barriers to allowing many of us to be able, whilst barriers in the environment cause many problems for many people. Others found barriers in the organisation of our society. The recognition of the many barriers did a lot to create a view of disability that many of the students had never considered before. There arose a great debate as an awareness of the real cause of disability became obvious.

Students were then asked about their experiences at the reception desk on their arrival at the hotel earlier today. Tim was the first to respond:

'Well, I'm feeling annoyed. From what we've discussed in this room up until now, I realise I blame myself and I apologise too much. I couldn't see to lip-read in reception and I'd no idea what the woman was saying to me and I apologised and then you came over, Alan, and I thought you were rude. I couldn't see what you were saying but I felt the atmosphere. Then the man took me in the office where it was well-lit and I felt I was a nuisance. But now I realise it's not my fault and I should have said to the receptionist, "I need to see your lips because I lip-read and the lighting is useless and you need to look at me when you speak to me".'

Someone from the group responded by asking Tim if he had the confidence to challenge as he was suggesting. And Tim responded firmly, 'No, you're right. But after our discussions, I think I may have in future. Alan's right. I've been thinking of myself as a second-class citizen but I realise I must change my thinking. We've only just begun the course and already I can see I need to change!'

Encouraging comments!

Stella was the next to speak: 'I thought I was a positive person but from what's been said this afternoon, I could be a lot better. I don't know about you lot but I could go home now and feel I'd gained already from the course!'

At this point, Peter fell from his chair in an epileptic seizure and we abandoned training. I dealt with Peter whilst Kathleen took over the rest of the group and directed them to the bar area where they could at least get refreshments.

Obviously everyone was a little shaken by Peter's episode and after I had got him to his room to rest awhile, I went to find the rest of the group to assure them that Peter was alright and to explain about epilepsy and how others might react to it. I didn't want any student to be scared and, most of all, I wanted Peter to be included in the group.

The whole group sat together for dinner that evening. No one separated themselves. I thought the group had bonded well and that was good but it did mean that Kathleen and I were involved with students at all times!

We had a rather energetic atmosphere in the training room the following

150

morning and everyone wanted to respond to my first question of the day.

'Tell me about yesterday? What did you learn? How do you feel? But before we go on, I want to speak to Peter! Peter, I really need you to know that I haven't broken your confidence. I haven't told anyone you have epilepsy!'

We all laughed together and Peter was laughing too! Many individuals in the group had positive comments about what they had learned from the training yesterday. The majority contributed to the notion: if you don't think positive about yourself, how can we expect others to feel positive about who we are? The other issue running through our discussion was that before the course they hadn't been aware of how many barriers each had to face daily.

Many of the students realised that they had been blaming themselves for so many things when actually it was the attitudes of others, the environmental design and the way society was organised (systems, services, policies and practices) which actually cause 'disability', rather than a person's medical diagnosis.

I think Tim reinforced the learning from yesterday by saying that if the reception had better lighting, he would have managed to lip-read and he would not have felt such an idiot!

This first session of the second day concluded by the group agreeing to a statement: 'By removing the barrier, you nearly always, remove disability!'

There are incidents that happen in everyone's life that are emotionally traumatic, so much so that they are never forgotten but are locked away in our subconscious and affect our thinking, our behaviour and our confidence when we least expect it. I really want my students to understand, and to accomplish that understanding, I related an experience from my own life to illustrate:

I was working in the garden in the front of our home. I was about 50 years of age at the time. Four young lads appeared at the bottom of the cul-de-sac where we lived and they proceeded to walk towards me. I estimated their ages to be between 9-11 years and they were laughing and seemed really happy. As they got nearer and nearer to me, a great fear came over me; I ran indoors, peered through the window and resumed my work in the garden when they had gone!

The question to the students was:

'Why do you think I behaved as I did? I had been teaching children for twenty-five years, so why should I be scared of four young boys? Why did I run away and hide?'

151

Fear is something each of us experience at some time in our lives and is an emotion that can override logic and common sense. Much of my fear is based on past experiences, usually from my childhood, when I would be ridiculed and taunted by other children. Or made to feel inadequate and inferior by professionals!

It was through working in the hospital service in my middle 20s that I overcame my fear of 'white coats'. So much did medical professionals mess with my head in my formative years that, for years, the sight of a person in a white coat would paralyse me! I say that I've overcome my fear but if I'm honest, even today there are residual issues and I would and do react to anyone wearing a white coat in a medical environment. Now I react defensively if not aggressively. Thankfully, medical personnel today do not seem to wear white coats whereas when I was a child, everyone in the hospital service wore a white coat!

We had lots of discussion on my 'flight' from the young lads walking up the street towards me and many people analysed the situation, but the real explanation was that the four boys laughing and walking towards me triggered memories from my childhood, when other children would laugh at me and ridicule me. Laugh at my speech. Laugh at my walking, laugh at my appearance. These incidents happened daily and were excruciatingly embarrassing and somehow, in an unguarded moment, I reverted back to childhood and past experiences and ran, thinking that the four lads might speak to me and ridicule and laugh.

The question was: 'Am I the only one who is affected by the past?'

Amazingly, everyone in the group had a story to tell! One woman student was really affected by this session. Through the discussion, she had realised that she reacted to her manager in a very negative way because he reminded her of a boyfriend who had jilted her years ago. She had not realised why she couldn't get on with her manager until discussion triggered her thinking. She became rather angry and stated, 'I've allowed this man to ruin my life! How could I do that and not really be aware of it?'

And so the discussion continued. Students became very aware of how negative past experiences affected them today.

The next session, the students had to discuss what past experiences triggered fear and how fear affected their lives. The atmosphere in the room during this discussion was electrifying. The students were absolutely animated. I allowed the discussion to go on for longer than the time scheduled on the programme as everyone was very involved. At the conclusion of the discussion, the comments were amazing! Each of the students seemed to be aware of how they reacted to past experiences and the element of fear they had in their lives.

One of our male students summed up the feelings of the group as he said, 'I realise now that I have allowed a lot of rubbish to enter my head regarding my condition and that rubbish has created fear and I react to that fear. Well, no more! I've discovered things about myself this morning that I never knew. I'm going to be far more positive when I go home!'

The majority of the group agreed but Stella seemed to be uncomfortable and I asked for her opinion.

'Oh Alan, you are a bugger! Why pick on me?'

'Stella, you seem to have gone quiet and I feel you have something to say that you're not saying.'

'Don't you miss anything? You're right as usual. I'm trying to hide away.'

'Come on now, lass. You can't hide away in here. Tell us what you're thinking.'

'What I'm thinking is personal to me. I don't think my thoughts apply to the rest of the group.'

'Well, now I think we are all intrigued so share your thoughts.'

'No, I don't want to bore people!'

'Stella, we are all interested. Tell us what you're thinking!'

The rest of the students encouraged and Stella became rather tearful. I felt so guilty for pressing her but then she began to speak.

'I'm sorry, folks. I'm just not used to my visual restrictions yet. The way you were all talking about fear just brought everything home to me. My sight changed four years ago. No one can explain how it happened or whether it will get better or deteriorate. So I live in constant fear. Each morning, I wake up and thank God that I still have the little bit of sight I have.'

Stella paused for breath and the room was quieted with the interest and anticipation.

Stella continued.

'Hearing you talking about fear made me realise how fearful I am all the time. I'm afraid to go out alone in case I bump into someone or something and hurt myself. I'm frightened that I might not see something in my path and fall over! I once fell down a hole about four feet deep. The workmen had left it momentarily to pack equipment in their van and along comes 'Calamity Jane' and down the hole I go. I don't know how it happened! I wasn't hurt, just a few scratches but I was so embarrassed, especially when three hefty workmen came to lift me out. That incident destroyed my confidence. I know I have a white stick and I've had mobility training but I'm still scared.'

There was a pause. The room was silent. The students seemed to be stunned and maybe there was empathy in the silence.

Stella seemed to take a few deep breaths as though she were composing herself, before continuing:

'Lots of people come to help me to cross a road. They see my white stick and they come to help. They will link their arm through mine or put my arm through theirs and I don't like it. They are complete strangers to me and they don't hesitate to touch me and I have no idea who they are; it's scary! Then there's my bloody husband. He comes home from work in the evening. Stops in the hallway to check the mail and take his coat and things off, then visits the bathroom, then the bedroom to take his tie off and then he comes to find me, usually in the kitchen, to tell me he is home. I hear him come in but even if I meet him in the hallway or by the front door I wouldn't know it was him until he spoke. When I hear him come in, I shout 'is that you?' but I never hear him reply. Every day I'm anxious. I hear him come in and I assume it's him. But it could be anyone. Why can't he come in and shout "I'm home" or "It's only me" before he checks the mail, etc.!'

Again, Stella pauses for breath and we all wait, not really knowing how to respond or even if Stella's finished.

'Talk about fear. Try eating out and not being able to see! Someone has to read the menu to me. But do you know not being able to see affects my hearing? I really have to concentrate on listening and there's always background noise in a restaurant. Then when I get my meal, I never know what's on my plate or where what is on my plate. If I ask for salt, someone will always give me the salt in my hand and I don't know if the salt comes out fast or how much is going on my food or where it's going on my plate or if I'm sprinkling salt on the table. Sometimes I don't know what I've got on my fork or what I'm putting into my mouth. Do you wonder I don't like going into a restaurant?'

I must admit to learning a lot from Stella's comments but I was at a loss to know how to respond to Stella. It was also interesting to hear other students with visual impairments agree with Stella and add their own stories.

'Thank you for sharing that, Stella,' I said, hastily trying to adjust my thoughts and get myself back on track. But there was more to come from Stella.

'Alan, do you mind if I say something else? After all, you did ask me to share my thoughts.'

I think most of the other students smiled at this comment and Stella took our attention once more.

'I don't want people to feel sorry for me. I have to live with my sight and I'm hoping to get used to it. It's still rather new to me. But I can't stop living because I can hardly see and this morning I've been made to think and I've learned that the way I react to fear can cause people to think I'm more of an oddity than I really am. For example, if the family want to go to a restaurant for a family meal and I say I don't want to go, I may be seen as being awkward or antisocial or even worse. So I'm learning to cope, learning strategies to overcome my fears. Alan, I hope you don't mind me saying this but the way you reacted to those boys when you were working in the garden could have made you even more vulnerable to ridicule!'

'Well, Stella. Thank you for that. Maybe you should come and stand where I am. I think you'd make a better trainer than I am.'

Addressing the group, I asked for comments on what had been said and the consensus of opinion was that we do need to be aware of how our past experiences affect our mind and our thinking. We do need to be aware of how negative thoughts and messages are linked to fear and how fear can affect our behaviour. People also realised how their potential had been blocked by negatives and fear.

Of course, Stella had to have the last word in this session:

'You know, folks, I've never talked about fear in my life before and I'm feeling really good. So maybe we need to talk more and when I go home, I'm going to find someone I can talk to. I think it might be quite liberating.'

I finished this session by explaining that in my opinion, everyone experiences fear at some time in their lives. For some people, it's an emotion that affects them daily. Some fears are understandable. But I need to be aware of the negative messages that I have internalised from my past that cause fear and hold me back.

During a short refreshment break, many of the students spoke of the effects the last session had had upon them and I was happy with the outcome.

The content of the rest of the course covered more positive topics. We looked at culture (lifestyle) and decided that 'disability is a culture' that the mainstream culture didn't accept, cater for or value and we discussed the implications of this; many students made positive and assertive plans for when they returned to work and indeed for their futures. Many agreed that by taking more control of their lives, they would reaffirm many positives.

Of course, Stella had regained her confidence and put the whole session into a nut shell:

'When I get back, I'm going to open my gob a lot more. I reckon I could do a lot more if I stopped comparing myself to the way I was before and start thinking "this is how I live now and this is how I do things"!'

Others followed Stella's lead and injected their own thoughts but the general opinion was that disability was a lifestyle and up until now they had tried to fit into mainstream and ignored their own individual lifestyle. The discussion continued and people remarked on how their aids and equipment, including wheelchairs, supported their lifestyle.

We then identified skills that each individual had. This was a really difficult session as people were either not aware of the skills they had or they were so modest, they didn't like to blow their own trumpet. However, through insistence on my part, each recognised they had many more skills than they thought. Then we discussed how many of our skills were developed and enhanced by our individual and unique lifestyles.

The conversations during breaks and at mealtimes had become much more positive and the majority of students seemed to be really enthusiastic.

As a result of our next group discussion, 'the positives of disability', people were ready and keen to participate. They quickly saw the reasoning behind this philosophy and the majority saw that there were many aspects of disability that were positive. Obviously, I was very quick to point out that some people had to live with pain or struggled to breath and many people might find it difficult to be positive about their lives but for the majority of students in the room at the time, there were positives that hadn't been identified before the course.

At the conclusion of the course, each student left with an action plan, parts of which were to be shared with their line manager. These action plans had been formulated through group discussions and personal tutorials with me. It was amazing to see how people had grown and developed over the period of the course. The group had bonded together and had supported each other so well that they seemed reluctant to say goodbye to each other. Each individual had a greater understanding of themselves and disability in general. At the beginning of the course, the majority of students blamed themselves for the many barriers that affected them and they were rather negative in defining their disabilities but we had laboured long and hard to illustrate the positives of disability. This concept of 'positives' was alien to all of the students at the beginning of the course. Now being aware of their skills and how their skills were often enhanced by their 'disability' had developed confidence, and that confidence added to personality, character and even charisma.

The evaluation and feedback I received at the end of the course was very encouraging and very positive. The course looked at my experiences of life. I shared the humorous and the embarrassing. I emphasised the positives of living with Cerebral Palsy. I shared the fears from my younger days; fears of not being able to work, fears of not getting married and having a family. I shared the transition from blaming myself to the realisation that 'society' caused me to be disabled rather than my medical label. It appeared that sharing my experiences and philosophies had transformed students' perceptions and made them more aware of who they really were. I was very sure that the course would have a strong and positive influence on their future lives and would inspire and encourage them to apply for relevant promotions!

I was really shocked at the outcomes. I was absolutely amazed that I could both design and deliver a course with such impact. I was ecstatic with my success as a trainer, for as the woman from the Job Centre had said a few years earlier, 'You have a speech impediment!' I was also immensely proud of Kathleen and of the way we had worked together. She had supported me really well throughout and it was such a good feeling to have her take some credit for, and share in the success of, the course.

CHAPTER TEN

There were a few things from the course I wanted to follow up on. I do have a 'mother hen' syndrome and I do tend to gather my chicks and succour them until I feel they are ready to leave the nest. I had concerns about two of my students; I really wanted to look into that which bothered me about them and support them through any problems they might have that hadn't been addressed on the course.

After speaking to the person in charge of my contract, I was introduced by telephone to their line managers.

Larry was about 35 years of age. He had joined the department at the age of 22 and worked as an audio typist. Larry lost his sight at the age of 17 due to a rather rare genetic condition that ultimately affected the optic nerve. A pre-course questionnaire revealed that Larry's line manager had concerns about the amount of time Larry had off from work on sickness leave. Certainly, Larry had to stay in bed for half a day during the course and I felt there were times during the course when Larry wasn't quite with it. Once or twice, he would be rather quiet and subdued. At times he would give inappropriate answers to questions. Often he would complain that the room was too hot (whilst the majority of others complained that they were chilly) and he would perspire and appear agitated. I noticed too that he drank quite a lot of water whilst in the classroom! He missed dinner on several evenings and said he had lain on his bed after class, gone to sleep and not woken until the following morning.

When I spoke to Larry about his health and his sickness record, he told me it was because of the genetic condition. Although I had nursing experience, I really did not understand Larry's explanation of his condition. I was really concerned as Larry said he had not seen his doctor for several years. Through his line manager, I was able to contact the department's occupational health team and they insisted that Larry saw his GP. Apparently, according to his GP, Larry's symptoms were all to do with his genetic condition! I was not surprised! Very often if one has a disability, every other ailment is attributed to it! However, I continued to talk with the occupational health team, who eventually arranged for Larry to have blood tests, which revealed diabetes and a problem in the liver. He was admitted to hospital and received appropriate treatment and medication.

After quite a time away from work on sick leave, Larry returned to work and his line manager reported that Larry was a new man. He was more energetic, more responsive and much more alert. An email from Larry to me confirmed that he hadn't felt so well for years and there was a little improvement in his eyesight too since he began treatment for diabetes. He thanked me for my perseverance as he believed his GP when he said his symptoms were part of his existing condition. I confess: I felt absolutely chuffed that I could have such an effect on someone's life.

The other student I was concerned about was a woman named Arleen. She was employed as an admin assistant and had been with the department for almost six years. I was surprised to find she was only 39 years of age. She looked considerably older! She had been very quiet throughout the course and had been quite aggressive when coaxed into participating. She didn't ever appear to smile and looked almost miserable! I found her behaviour rather odd. She never appeared for breakfast. Sometimes she would appear for mid-morning refreshments. Kathleen and I and several of the other students had noticed that Arleen seemed to visit the supermarket daily. The supermarket was a considerable drive away and there were many students who didn't have their cars with them, but never would Arleen offer anyone a ride, even if asked. In my opinion, she was a real loner! She sometimes appeared wobbly on her feet and she had a distinct hand tremor! On occasions, her speech appeared to be slurred and she seemed very lethargic. Kathleen and I had voiced our concerns to each other about Arleen since the first day of the course. Neither Kathleen nor I could make a relationship with her. I did ring her line manager because of her non-attendance in the mornings and I was told Arleen had been sent on the course with the manager hoping it would help sort her out because if she didn't change, she would be sacked. Her line manager had said Arleen had been a great worker until two years ago and suddenly she changed almost overnight.

I spoke with Arleen face-to-face in a one-to-one. Arleen's husband had walked out a year ago and Arleen lived alone in the marital home and said she found it really hard to cope. She also told me she had been diagnosed with fibromyalgia. She informed me that she found the content of the course a waste of time. She said she hadn't volunteered to come on the course but had been almost forced into coming by her line manager and senior manager.

My knowledge of fibromyalgia was non-existent but from Arleen's behaviour and physical manifestations, I thought it was something cerebral.

When I mentioned the condition to Kathleen, she said she had heard the term before but could not remember from where. As we were talking, I suddenly remembered. In the 1980s we had attended the Westminster conferences. These conferences were held monthly at the Westminster Hospital in London. They were organised and chaired by the resident professor of rheumatology and each month a different new diagnosis or other aspect of disability was discussed. These conferences were so interesting and I was sure fibromyalgia had been a topic for one of the conferences.

Kathleen phoned the Westminster Hospital and eventually spoke with the professor who sent us information by fax to the hotel.

According to the information received from the Professor, fibromyalgia was quite new and lots of research had been undertaken into the condition since the late 1970s. Apparently, fibromyalgia typically causes pain and tenderness in many areas of the body. This pain can be rather persistent and the severity of pain differs from person to person. Fibromyalgia also causes tiredness, which can be extreme in some cases. The information sent to us suggested that the condition was more common in women than in men.

The most interesting part of the information was about diagnosis. Diagnosis was by a doctor's examination. At the time (early 1990s) there were no laboratory tests to confirm the diagnosis! The professor stated that in his opinion, fibromyalgia was difficult to diagnose. He said he had many people said to have the condition attend his clinics, but fibromyalgia did not affect the joints as the rheumatic diseases did but affect the fibrous tissues, such as tendons and ligaments.

There was a theory at the time that the cause of the condition might involve changes to the brain's chemicals. I knew from my nursing experience that brain chemicals were important and there had to be a balance of chemicals in the brain to be healthy. These changes need only to be minute to stop the brain transmitting messages, in this case between nerve cells and the brain. So in my thinking at this time, I thought Arleen might be very sensitive to pain.

As I spoke with Arleen in the one-to-one situation, she was difficult to get to respond. The only information she gave me was that the course was a waste of her time and that she had fibromyalgia!

On my return home from the course, I contacted Arleen's line manager and gave my comments and assessments of Arleen whilst on the course. We had a lengthy discussion and the line manager had far more concerns than even I had. I learned a little more about Arleen's background. The line manager told me that Arleen had suffered a terrible breakdown about two and a half years ago and had spent several weeks in a psychiatric hospital. She had been away from work for six months on this occasion. Arleen returned to work and after about six weeks she began to complain of tiredness and aches and pains. Sometimes she would take two or three days off, sometimes she would leave work because the tiredness and the aches and pains got too much for her and sometimes she would turn up for work very late, maybe lunch time! So she had a very erratic work attendance. Previous to Arleen's breakdown, she had been a good and reliable worker, actually a model employee, and very popular with the office team. The line manager reported that there had been incidents in the office of heated confrontations caused by Arleen; money and other personal items had disappeared from handbags and desk drawers and although nothing could be proved, everyone suspected Arleen! Then came the break-up of her marriage. This affected Arleen and once again she became ill.

There had been many meetings involving the line manager, senior management and top management and they were loath to terminate Arleen's employment. It seemed to me that they were waiting and hoping the medical problems would improve and Arleen would return to her former self.

I was very surprised at the patience and tolerance of the department. In my opinion, the department was not a charity but a business! I was asked for my thought on the situation regarding Arleen by a very senior manager from human resources. My comments were based on the conversations I'd had with Arleen's line manager and my own observation of Arleen whilst she was on the course. They were:

Is it good business sense to retain Arleen in the present situation?

Is it good practice that public money is being used to pay Arleen's salary when her performance and attendance are far below what is expected of others?

Is it actually good for Arleen to 'get away' with her erratic attendance and behaviour?

Would some kind of disciplinary hearing, warning or even a disciplinary contract that Arleen would sign and consent to help to modify her behaviour and attendance?

Is the management of Arleen affected because of sympathy towards all that had happened to her?

Would stronger management help Arleen to modify her behaviour?

What effect does Arleen's situation have on the rest of the team who work in the office with her?

At this time, we were looking forward to and preparing for the implementation of the Disability Discrimination Act and I suspect that this had a bearing on the department's tolerance of Arleen.

My recommendations were that, with Arleen's permission, a case conference was arranged, including management, occupational health, Arleen's GP and her psychiatrist.

As per usual in those days, I was very busy to check on how my comments had been received and after my initial conversation with human resources I didn't hear anything for a considerable time.

It was on one of my infrequent rest days that I rang for news of Arleen. Her line manager had consulted with her to gain permission to hold a case conference but Arleen would not give permission and had not been seen since! Letters had been sent to her home but no reply had been made. Visits had been made to her home but no one ever answered the door.

I was told every attempt to contact Arleen had failed. The legal team for the department had been involved and Arleen's employment had been terminated as a result of sixteen weeks nonattendance and failure to reply to departmental correspondence and supply a medical certificate for the period of absence from work!

My work with the department continued and it was on the fourth training course I did for managers that I actually met Arleen's line manager. On enquiring about Arleen, I was told how Arleen had been found sleeping rough – it was said she was addicted to alcohol – and was now on a psychiatric ward in a secure prison, awaiting trial for theft! I was devastated. Had my recommendation thrown her over the edge? I was really concerned about my actions in all of this. Why had I not picked up on how serious Arleen's condition had been whilst she had been on the course? Of course, when I applied reasoning to my emotional questioning I realised that I had only known Arleen for the short duration of the course; others had known her longer and saw her almost daily and if her GP and her Psychiatrist had not been able to foresee the future for Arleen, I had no cause to beat myself up.

To be truthful, I do get involved with my students. Each individual is important to me. I like to see their progress. I share their joys and their sorrows. I have a genuine interest in each of them and maybe this adds to the success of my training. I have been involved with so many who have acquired disability and to say their lot is difficult is an understatement. I do wonder if Arleen's acquired condition contributed to her breakdown, or was it the problems in her marriage or maybe a combination of both? I'll never know! I wonder too if the slurred speech, the hand tremors and the unsteady walking were to do with her drinking and I hadn't picked up on that either. What about her trips to the supermarket? Always, she went alone, almost secretively. But I cannot be responsible for students' behaviour outside of the training room!

The training courses for managers were always interesting and very popular. We had a waiting list of people wanting to attend and so the department arranged more courses to meet the demand. The content of these courses was threefold.

The first and foremost purpose of the course was to explain the programme for the personal development course that employees with disabilities attended; they were managed by people attending the managers' course and had to explain and discuss action plans presented to line managers by the employees who had completed the personal development course.

The second phase of the course was to present and discuss certain items from the Disability Discrimination Act. We discussed and dissected the 'definition of disability' as contained in the act, as the department saw the understanding of the definition as crucial to the implementation of the act. There really wasn't a great deal of time in the one day programme to spend too much time on the act. Clients other than the department were commissioning me to deliver two and three-day training events on the act!

Always, on the managers' course, there was interest and lots of discussion on 'reasonable adjustment', which in my opinion was an important and central part of the act. I saw the clause on 'reasonable adjustment' as the most liberating part of the new act for employees with disability. I always laboured the implications of this part of the act.

I would quote from the clause on reasonable adjustment as it appeared in the act and the managers would discuss what was needed to implement the principles and concepts into their daily responsibilities. The act stated:

'The concept of reasonable adjustment arises where the nature of a disability creates the need for a job to be done in a different way.'

Another statement from the act was:

'Since the effect of disability varies from person to person the required adjustment will vary accordingly.'

By taking this clause from the act stage by stage rather than introducing it as a whole, I believed there was more learning and certainly more discussion. The final quote was also received with interest and speculation:

'The duty to make reasonable adjustment means that a potential employer cannot say that a particular individual is unsuitable for a job (or a promotion) because of certain aspects of his or her disability where reasonable adjustment would have eliminated the problem.'

I took the liberty of inserting the words (or a promotion) because the major reason for my work with the department was to prepare employees with disability for promotion and get them to rise in the organisation of the department.

The third phase of the managers' course was for them to ask questions regarding the employees they managed and to discuss the best possible practice for managing employees with disability.

A managers' course never finished on time! There seemed to be so much interest and discussion. The majority of managers really took their responsibilities seriously and were so engaged as to ask for an extension to the day.

A group of managers who worked in the same geographical area got together after they had attended the day's course, created a document and published it on the intranet to invite comments from other employees.

The document was headed 'Suggested Steps to Remove Disability Discrimination.'

There were eleven suggestions contained in the document and I knew when I saw it that if the steps became practice, the plight of disabled employees would drastically change for the better. The suggestions were:

Know the law.

Provide definitions of discrimination, bullying, harassment, etc.

Make all staff aware of their role in maintaining an inclusive environment.

Create inclusive policies.

Identify and remove all barriers that cause disability.

Remove barriers to individuals reporting discrimination, etc.

Consult with disabled employees and others in the community.

Gain and ensure senior management support for initiatives.

Train all staff in disability equality and diversity.

Communicate the Departments position in promoting disability equality and diversity.

Monitor, evaluate and report the effectiveness of policies, practices and procedures.

***

Sometimes I had to pinch myself to make sure I was experiencing reality. I found it absolutely incredible that I could influence people through my training so much that a very large central government department could take on change and adapt and adopt policies, practices and procedures to accommodate and value disabled people. I know at this time that disability was on the political agenda as employers prepared for the implementation of the Disability Discrimination Act but for me to learn of senior managers using their own time, outside of working hours, to consider and debate issues raised by me in the training room was awe-inspiring.

I cannot forget certain experiences from my earlier life. I was given awful and negative messages and I was led to believe that I wouldn't attain very much in life.

The powers that be had tried to label me as a mentally defective. My parents were told that I would be uneducable and that I would never walk or talk. It was recommended that my right arm be amputated because a false arm would be of more use to me. I had been told that I would never work, earn my living, never marry or have children and I had been told my speech was so awful, I would never earn my living as a trainer. Well, is it any wonder that I felt a remarkable and powerful sense of achievement!? Here I was, working with some of the highest in the land and influencing Central Government Departments. I did wonder at this ecstatic time in my life whether my life would have been so exciting and rewarding if I had have been born without cerebral palsy?

And through all of this, I was infinitely aware of working alongside Kathleen. We were together twenty-four hours a day, seven days a week and we got on so well. We travelled extensively! Many times we were on the road at 5:30 in the morning. Often we wouldn't get home until ten in the evening and we would be up and off again the next morning. It might be important to say here that I don't think life was easy for Kathleen. It took me at least an hour to shave, shower and dress. I would need help with the odd shirt button and cuff links, etc., and Kathleen was always there. Others may take ten minutes to get ready. It wasn't possible for Kathleen or me to lie in bed until the last minute. I'm sure living with me requires the other person to have patience! Kathleen has always had that required patience. We work together as one! We often worked five days a week and often stayed in hotels. The pace was relentless and we had to be really organised. I know many wives who would have complained, but not Kathleen; she was there for me. We had a wonderful relationship, (still have) and I adore her. It is such a privilege to have such a wonderful and compatible companion! Kathleen sustained me, supported and encouraged me in setting up Focus disABILITY. She always had time to help me sort out teething problems and if I wavered in believing in myself or believing in my abilities as an entrepreneur, she would administer a metaphorical boot up the backside and an injection of confidence. Kathleen is an angel sent from Heaven to help prepare us for something wonderful. I don't really know what that something is. I only know that as Kathleen and I travel hand in hand through this world, life becomes increasingly wonderful! Whenever I'm with Kathleen, life becomes exciting. Many have contributed to my life but Kathleen, my wise and wonderful wife, made me the man I am! She is an essential part of me and a vital part of my life!

I would love to meet those people from my past who reinforced negatives and gave me such a hard time. Those people who put me down and had such low expectations of me. They made me feel a freak, destroyed my self-worth and restricted my growth, development and confidence! I can only say, 'come the revolution, certain people are mine, so hands off!' On the contrary, though, I'm sure that exposure to the 'bad guys' helped make me strong and determined and gave me whatever one needs to cope. That exposure also greatly heightened the sense of any achievement and gave credence to my mantra 'We'll show the buggers!'

Starting my own business was not really planned. It became necessary as a means of paying a mortgage and supporting a family. My business didn't come from any desire to change the world or the plight of disabled people. I had very little knowledge of the issues involved in 'disability' before I launched myself on the world as a trainer. I had my autobiography published in 1982, I had appeared on numerous television shows and I used my 'media exposure' to gain entry into establishments to promote Focus disABILITY. I seemed to do well but in retrospect, I wonder if sometimes fate will take one by the hand and lead one somewhere without one even realising it. It's only when one looks back that one notices. Many may call it the hand of the Lord! It had taken a little more than two years to establish myself as a trainer and develop a good, solid and reliable clientele. I had so much work coming in that I was able to contract some of it out to other disabled trainers.

I felt I was a success inasmuch as my motivation in setting up my business was to pay the mortgage and support my family and I was certainly doing that.

Always have I been told that necessity is the mother of invention but for me, responsibility is the stimulator of necessity! I'm not too sure that my mortgage and my family responsibilities were the only source of wind under my wings! I liked the buzz I received from my work and the whole family enjoyed the fruits of my labour, for we had surplus after we had met all our monthly financial requirements. I had to earn in order to support and in earning, I enjoyed achieving and the development and the discovery of talents and skills I never knew I had.

Also, as my awareness of the issues around disability grew, so did my desire to promote equality and awareness. I became an ambassador and a more militant representative of both the political and secular elements of disability. I was also able to help others through my newfound knowledge and through the use of my counselling skills. I enjoyed this element of my work; it gave me job satisfaction.

As it became obvious that my business was a success, there were people who seemed not to want me to succeed. I asked myself why certain people were sceptical and scathing about my work and ambition, and I found it difficult to believe that anyone would want me to crash and fail. It was as though they thought that I should not attract affluence because in their eyes I was a disabled person. I developed a theory. I suspected there were people out there who lacked the courage to go out and make a difference to their own lives and to the lives of others, whereas I, who in their eyes, was an inferior being, had accomplished what they couldn't. I developed my courage through the experience of living with cerebral palsy. I like who I am and my disability adds to my ability!

I'm sure the success in running my business made some other people feel mediocre! So-called friends would make comments like, 'You can't run a business from your address, you need a bigger and more prestigious address', or 'You're really wasting your time. I know so many people who have tried to run their own business and failed! Or 'I know people who have lost money and friends'.

I really had to ask myself, were these negative comments being hurled at me to stop me succeeding? All justified expressing such thoughts by saying, 'I'm not trying to be hurtful! I'm just trying to spare you the pain of failure!' I thought it ironic that comments like these should be expressed after I had secured contracts and after success was obvious.

The reality of the situation was that these people just opened their mouths and exposed their own limitations. They hadn't done their homework. They had no idea of how many bookings I had in my diary or how many long-term contracts I had. I wondered too if my success made them feel a failure! I'm sure it was obvious to all that after experiencing our bad times, my illness and my retiring from teaching and all that went with it, Kathleen and I were prospering and actually living a dream. I too wondered if non-disabled people who were successful had such comments hurled at them!

Of course, I knew the origins of all the negatives. In general terms, society is obsessed with appearances! They think one has got to look good in order to be a success; well in my case, one has got to have guts and integrity in order to win!

People other than my immediate family had no idea of how hard I worked to achieve recognition as a trainer, nor had they any inkling of the stress and worry I endured in the early days of business.

Success is individual to everyone! I felt good about myself. I felt strong and healthy. I was confident and happy in my relationship with Kathleen. My family were happy. There were no contentions in my home and I was able to support my family physically, financially and emotionally. Whenever I wasn't working, I enjoyed being at home and I had enough work to keep me going for the considerable future. All of these things meant success to me! I measure success in terms of my family being united and happy. Success in business, for me, is the ability to recognise opportunity, take it and run with it. I had developed strategies of coping in order to seize and take advantage of each opportunity that presented itself to me.

I had identified goals at the start of my business; most of these goals were achieved as I progressed in business and these goals helped me measure success. Maybe the fact that most of these goals were family-oriented encouraged and motivated a strong enthusiasm to achieve. Nevertheless, I developed. As I changed from a teacher to an entrepreneur, I became aware of my shortcomings (which others might call shyness or a lack of confidence) and I had to overcome them and strengthen the inner man. I was really proud of how well I was doing and nothing breeds success like success. Nothing breeds confidence, either, like success.

Since beginning work as a trainer, I had been concerned about paying bills and supporting my wife and family but of a sudden, I felt differently as to why I was working. I felt I was now offering a service that was useful to the cause of disability but also aided the development of individuals who attended my courses. It was still important for me to earn in order to keep our home together but my business became more of a vocation and much more rewarding than a fund raiser, inasmuch as I felt qualified for all that I did by my experience; undoubtedly, my academic qualifications helped with presentation skills but it was the experience of living with cerebral palsy in a world geared to non-disabled people that had contributed, more than anything else, to my innate dedication to counsel and care for the development of delegates and students.

CHAPTER ELEVEN

Travelling the country and being involved with training meant that I met many disabled people, some of whom became my friends, and I discovered life can be fun, even hilarious when you mix with such friends!

I was commissioned to chair a conference in Edinburgh for the European Commission. The conference was to compare services offered in each of the represented countries for disabled people and one of my friends, who acquired a problem with his sight, had a slot on the programme. He had been registered blind some eight months before the course and was adjusting to a new style of living. He wouldn't normally have travelled alone but I promised to be on the same train and look out for him at his station. He used a white cane and the general public were ordinarily kind and helpful! He was anxious about staying in a hotel room on his own and there were a great many first-time experiences for him on this trip. I met him as planned and all went well.

We briefly met with all the delegates who were from various countries within the EU and we also met with four interpreters who were going to interpret the proceedings of the three-day conference into different languages to accommodate our foreign guests. It was a brief session just to welcome and introduce everyone, discuss a few domestics and orientate people around the hotel. For me it was an opportunity to allow people to tune into my speech and to get rid of any anxiety I may have had. I always feel better after my first contact with a group on each commission I receive!

My friend stayed by my side as much as possible throughout this first meeting and I could understand his lack of confidence. As is my usual practice, I invited anyone with any facilitation needs to make them known and, amongst others, two people came forward also using white sticks. One man and one woman, and although they both came from different countries, they each spoke

English. They quickly struck up a rapport with my friend and arranged to meet for dinner.

At the dinner table, I had to read the menu and I was very aware that I was alone with three blind people who all needed my attention. When the food arrived, they needed to know what was on their plates and where it was. Luckily I knew the procedure from past experience: potatoes at two o'clock, meat at six o'clock, etc., but because there were three of them and because there was a great deal of background noise in the dining room with everyone chatting, I had to be sure that each individual knew I was talking to them. Sometimes conversation can be really confusing when one cannot see, particularly if there's lots of background noise! People sitting at adjacent tables were speaking to us as well and this caused distraction. I think this might have been the cause of the problem!

My fellow diner sitting on my left touched my arm to make sure he had my attention and asked, 'Is your meat tough? I can't cut through mine! I may have to send it back!'

When I looked, I had to inform him that he was actually trying to cut through his tie, which had flopped on top of his meat. I assumed this had happened when he had turned to speak to someone behind him! It caused the four of us to laugh but I'm not sure others around us understood the situation as one cannot see a visual impairment without the mobility aid of a white cane or guide dog!

***

The three days of conference were busy for me but I shared the same table with my three friends each meal time and we got to know each other really well. I suppose it was inevitable that we shared a taxi to the railway station at the end of conference! So I found myself at Edinburgh station with three blind people and I had to be their eyes. We all linked arms and proceeded to walk to the station forecourt to look at the information board. There we stood, arms linked: three men and one woman and three white sticks, each with baggage over our shoulders as well! Suddenly we were confronted by a middle-aged and rotund woman who demanded in a broad Scottish accent:

'Where are you going?'

'It's alright,' I said. 'I can see!'

'I know you can, dearie! But I can see better!'

172

'No, you misunderstand. I can see well!'

'Oh, maybe so but you still need my help. I know you do! The spirits communicated with me this morning and told me to come early for my train because I'd be needed and I received a vision of four people with white sticks!'

It was obvious that this woman was not going to be deterred, and taking her place in the middle of the line, a man linked with the woman's left arm and two white sticks while me and my friend linked to her right arm and one white stick; we were guided by a woman with a brilliantly gleaming face to our train!

I'm sure it was obvious to all who saw us that this woman had a mission to fulfil. No words were needed! Her deportment, her bearing, her stride and her facial expression said it all!

I felt we were making her day!

We had discovered that we could all take the same train provided it stopped at relevant stops on the way.

We found our train but the woman's mission was not complete. She would not allow us to get on the train until she had found the guard and introduced us to him as 'four very special people'. It didn't end there! Our specialness was further emphasised by the woman's parting comment to the guard:

'Look after them well. They are so, so special, otherwise I would not have received my communication and vision from the world of spirits this morning! Someone who has gone before is watching over them!'

After we were seated on the train and when we were sure the woman had gone, all four of us collapsed into uncontrollable laughing. We weren't laughing at the woman's religious beliefs – more at the way she 'helped' us and the way she made us feel!

We were entertained for the rest of our journey together as we debated who was the more special and why!

***

I was concerned about the amount of time Kathleen was spending away from home as my P.A. on training courses. Not that she ever complained but I knew she liked to look after the home and cook and look after us all as a family.

We discussed options as a family and fortunately, I was able to employ other disabled people to accompany me on day-long training courses to allow Kathleen days at home to catch up on office work or domestic chores. All the people I employed were employed on a casual basis. Kathleen was still my main and preferred P.A. and worked with me on residential courses.

Early one morning, I embarked on a never-to-be-forgotten journey. On this particular morning I had a man travelling with me who I employed as a personal assistant. He had been a photographer for a national newspaper and had contracted some medical condition that affected his eyes and his sight. He had already lost one eye and the sight in his other eye was deteriorating. He was no longer able to follow his career as a photographer but he had sufficient sight to enable him to write on a flip chart and to do all the other tasks I needed him to do to support me in the training room.

We left my home just before dawn and I took a countrified route to avoid the often busy motorways. As I drove along, we witnessed the splendour of a sunrise with the trees silhouetted against a beautiful flaming red sky and we wondered with awe at the amazing sights that surrounded us.

As we were travelling along a rather quiet country road, a car overtook me at some considerable speed, quite near to a bend in the road! I personally thought how dangerous it was to overtake at that point in the road. The driver of the other vehicle travelled quite some distance on the wrong side of the road and found a motorbike in his path. They both swerved to avoid each other. The car hit a tree head-on, on my side of the road, and the motorcyclist was thrown over the front of his bike as his front wheel hit the high kerb on his side of the road.

I have nursing experience and I have first aid training, but I felt rather scared and debated with myself if I should involve myself with the accident. The big question was: how would I feel tomorrow or in the future if I just drove on?

So I stopped my car and didn't know who to attend to first. My companion in the passenger seat was hysterical and frozen; I couldn't even get him to get out of the car so I had no choice but to administer a hefty slap around his face. I shook him into some semblance of coherence and demanded that he phone the emergency services. I did have concerns about how the casualties might react to me but I really had to forget myself. I needed to be strong for others. I ran over to the motorcyclist and, as calmly as I could, asked where he was hurt and got very little response. So I asked if he would lie still and not remove his helmet. He was lying on his back and I didn't know if he had landed in that position when he had been thrown over the handlebars of his motorcycle or whether he had moved into that position himself, but I didn't want him to move again. I repeated that I didn't want him to move or remove his helmet and the expression on his face conveyed to me that he understood. I then ran over to the driver of the car, checking with my PA that the emergency services had been called and I was assured they had. My PA then went to the back of my car and proceeded to vomit.

As I approached the other car, the driver had his seatbelt off and the car door opened and was trying to get out. I quickly called to him and told him to stay where he was. There was steam and a hissing sound coming from the front of the car where it had impacted on the tree. In trepidation I walked around the car looking and smelling for leaking petrol. I was quite certain there was no petrol leaking so with mounting apprehension I turned my attention to the driver. I said, 'I'm a first aider and I can see your leg is damaged and bleeding. Are you hurt anywhere else?' I could see absolute terror in his eyes. I could feel his attitude towards me. Maybe I could understand his reaction but this man needed my help! Having a disability does not stop one being concerned for his fellow men.

I once again asked, 'Are you hurt any where else other than your leg?' To which he replied in rather a loud voice, 'Get away. Get away. You're a bloody loony!' I didn't really know what to do! Maybe I was wrong in thinking it was my disability he was reacting to. I'm sure I can be over sensitive and misread situations. This guy might have reacted to anyone. He was in shock and maybe he felt vulnerable, or was he reacting to my impeded speech? Removing my tie, I advised the driver to remain in his seat and said, 'I'm going to put my tie around your upper leg and use it as a tourniquet because your lower leg is bleeding heavily.'

He became rather agitated, told me to bugger off and once again called me a loony! I really had no option. The man was bleeding profusely and I didn't quite know where from. His right trouser leg below the knee was saturated with blood and there was a pool of blood on the floor of the car. I proceeded to put my tie around his upper leg whilst he beat me on my shoulders and upper arms with his fists. I was concerned. The airbag in his car had gone off, which had protected his upper body on impact but I would rather have had him sitting still in his seat. I did not know whether his neck or back had been damaged and whether the blows he was raining on me might make any possible damage worse! The blows subsided a little and then the driver vomited down the back of my shirt. I managed to put my tie around his upper leg and pulled it as tight as I could, at the same time explaining once again that I hoped it would stem the flow of blood! Unless I uncovered the wound, I could not tell if I had stopped or lessened the bleeding. The driver was so distressed. I did not want to add to it by tearing his trouser leg to reveal the wound. I was hoping the emergency services would soon arrive! The driver became aggressive and abusive once again and I'm afraid I retaliated.

'Look, mate!' I said, 'I'm the only person here who can help you at the moment. I cannot help my speech! It's been like this all my life. There is nothing wrong with my brain or intellect. I assure you, I know what I'm doing! I want you to sit as still as you can in case you've damaged your neck or your spine! Do not touch or loosen my tie which is around your leg. You may have damaged an artery. You're bleeding heavily. My tie is really tight around your leg to stop the bleeding. Leave it alone. I'm going to look at the driver of the motorcycle. I'll be back to loosen the tourniquet shortly. Do you understand?'

I could not do anymore for him and I thought if I removed myself from his presence he might have become less agitated.

Obviously the man was distressed. He was also verbally aggressive and made it very clear that he thought I was a 'nutcase'. He broke down in floods of tears and moved to exit the car. I had to restrain him and once again explained to him about my speech. I told him an ambulance would soon arrive and explained my concern about possible damage to his neck and spine. His frustration with me was so obvious!

There was no one else around. No other vehicle had passed the scene since the accident so I was entirely on my own.

My travelling companion was rendered absolutely useless from the shock of it all. I restrained the driver in his seat by replacing his seat belt and tying it to the rear seat belt, explaining why I was doing it and that I hoped the emergency services would soon arrive.

I did feel pangs of conscience in tying the driver to his seat but as he would not heed what I asked and because I was concerned that he might have injured his spine or neck, it really was for his own good!

The motorcyclist was really dazed and I did not want him to lose consciousness so I asked a lot of questions and kept him talking. He was twenty-one years of age. He worked the night shift in a large warehouse as a picker. He had finished work at around 6:30 that morning and had travelled a rather short distance before the accident. He was travelling to see his girlfriend in the next town, hoping to see her before she left for work. I got his girlfriend's name and telephone number, hoping I could remember them should the rider lose consciousness before the emergency services arrived.

Eventually the police and the ambulance arrived almost simultaneously. I was so relieved! I explained to the ambulance personnel what I had done and why and what time I had applied the tourniquet to the car driver's leg.

The ambulance man went to the car driver whilst the ambulance woman went to the motor cyclist. One of the policemen also went over to the

176

motorcyclist.

The other policeman spoke to my companion but then came over to me and asked me to walk with him to the crashed car. I could understand why: I thought two casualties, two ambulance people – two policemen to assist, one with each casualty! As we approached the car, I heard the driver say to the ambulance man, 'Thank god you're here! Someone normal at last! Please keep that cretin away from me! He put that on my leg and he made it worse. It really hurts and he's fastened me in my seat. I can't get out! The bastard!'

The ambulance man assured him that I had done all the right things and asked him to sit as still as possible. He put a supportive collar around the driver's neck and administered oxygen. He then asked the policeman, who was talking to me, to make sure his colleague was okay and to bring a spinal board from the ambulance. The policeman asked me to stay where I was and went over to the motorcyclist to do as he had been asked.

The casualties were eventually put into the ambulance and driven away. I was exhausted and suffering from shock and suddenly concerned that I was now going to be very late for the training day. It was too early in the morning to call my client and I really was in an awful state physically and appearance-wise. My shirt sleeves were covered in blood and the back of my shirt was covered in vomit!

My companion and I were detained by the police anyway because they wanted to question us and help them with their report. I was really smelly and needed to sit in my car so I looked in the boot of my car and fortunately found a roll of black bin bags. I protected my seat and sat in the car. Within seconds, a police officer appeared, thrust open the driver's door and snatched the keys from the ignition whilst informing me, rather aggressively, 'You're not going anywhere, sunshine. Just wait there!'

I really had no intention of going anywhere. I just needed to sit quietly for a short time to recover from the tension and the shock of dealing with the two casualties.

I can usually cope with any emergency with efficiency but when the emergency is over and I've dealt with it, I experience a reaction and need a little time to recover!

My companion had been taken to the police car and was sat in the front passenger seat talking to a police officer. Eventually the police officer came and sat in the passenger seat of my car and asked for my driving licence and insurance. It was obvious, from his first questions, that he thought I had been involved in the accident, if not the cause of it!

I became very assertive and defensive and quickly recited all that had happened.

At the conclusion of my account, he looked at me and said, 'You did all that. I'm amazed. You don't look like you could do any of that!'

That one comment was 'the straw that broke the camel's back'. My hackles began to rise and in my anger I retorted, 'I think I've had enough this morning! I've been sworn at, called names, beaten, vomited on and now I don't know whether you are being patronising or just plain rude. I don't think you should make any assumptions about what I can or cannot do based on my appearance!' He just looked at me in arrogance and said, 'I just need a factual report!'

After going over the details of the accident again, I was then asked to wait. My mind was beginning to focus on what I should do about my client, who was expecting me to facilitate a training day for his staff later that morning. As always, when in trouble, phone the wife!

I could not find my mobile and realised my companion had it. I got out of my car and proceeded to walk towards the police car to ask for my mobile, only to be confronted by the police officer who demanded I get back in my car. I explained that I needed my mobile phone and he completely ignored what I was saying and quite rudely demanded I get back in my car!

I did as I was told but I was seething! The other officer eventually approached my car and sat by my side. 'Are you alright?' he asked. 'Your mate has been telling me what you did for those two fellows this morning.' He was older than the other officer and seemed much more polite.

'I am okay, thank you. My mate has my mobile phone and I would like to make a call. I'm on my way to work and the accident has delayed me and I need to let people know I'm going to be very late.'

'There's no problem there but let me make that call for you!'

I explained that I wanted to phone my wife, who would inform my client and organise everything for me. I explained that I needed to stop off somewhere and buy a new shirt and tie and possibly find somewhere to have a shower.

'No problem!' he said and walked away with the telephone number to ring Kathleen.

I was still perturbed. I needed my mobile. I needed Kathleen to call me back and tell me what she had arranged with my client. I think, too, I needed to speak to Kathleen, for I am sure I would have found the comfort I needed in just hearing her voice!

After a time, the older officer returned and said he had phoned Kathleen and he had also phoned the company I was working for that day and the training course had been postponed and would be rebooked.

We were finally escorted to the local police station. The older officer bought me a shirt on the way and arranged for me to have a shower at the station too! Eventually, we were asked to sign a statement and given news of the two men injured in the accident.

Apparently, the driver of the car had punctured a main artery behind the knee of his right leg as well as damaging his knee and had several broken bones in his right leg. It was suggested that the movement of the driver trying to leave the car had caused the broken bones to puncture the artery. By all accounts, I was right in applying my tie as a tourniquet and telling him to sit still and stay in the car! The motorcyclist was said to have mild concussion!

The attitude of the driver towards me as I tried to help him in his hour of need had upset me to some extent. I don't go around thinking of how my disability affects my appearance and it's always like a slap in the face when others react to me as though I were an alien. I don't hear my impeded speech! When I speak, I hear the words very clearly in my head!

Occasions like this always get me down somewhat but I cannot allow the thoughts, feelings and actions of others to have a negative effect on me. Why should I feel guilty about something I cannot help? I have to remain confident, for my image and behaviour are an example to others. I also have a wife and family at home and I have a very strong sense of responsibility towards them, which lifts me from any gloom or negativity.

In my opinion, I did well in coping with all the results of the accident. Maybe better than many others! I also had battle scars! My upper left arm and back were really bruised where the driver had punched me. I could not wait to get home to Kathleen, for in her company I find solace, soothing and total acceptance.

I considered myself to be very fortunate as I continued in business. I never advertised or needed to go into cold calling. Bookings came my way through recommendations based on reputation. The contracts I had with central government departments continued, although I had to tender to renew the contracts each year. Nevertheless, my work with government departments increased.

***

Positivity is my middle name. I love life and live it to the full but I must confess that I become angry whenever I am patronised or reminded of my differences.

Kathleen and I were shopping in a large superstore and my shoelace had come undone so just like other people, I stopped and crouched to retie it. The way I tie my shoelaces may look awkward and difficult to the onlooker but for me, it's the only way I can do it and I'm used to it.

As I was crouched tying my shoe, Kathleen carried on looking at goods on the shelves. One of the shop assistants, an older woman, who looked over retirement age, took Kathleen by the arm and, pointing at me, said:

'Shouldn't you be doing that for him? He's struggling!'

Kathleen replied, 'Don't worry. He can manage.'

'But as his carer, aren't you paid to do things like that for him?'

At this point, I re-joined Kathleen and asked if anything was wrong.

'Nothing wrong, dear, just people making gross assumptions! Come on, let's move away.'

Kathleen took my arm and we walked to another part of the store, away from the offending assistant, and Kathleen continued to shop.

Eventually, we took our purchases to the pay desk and the offending assistant was the only member of staff on the till. Kathleen placed her goods on the counter and then discovered she hadn't got her credit card in her handbag so we had to use mine!

(This was at the time when Chip and PIN was quite new.) I presented my card to the assistant for payment and requested that I sign, rather than use my PIN.

The assistant looked at me with her head held to one side, as though I were an adorable little puppy dog, and announced, 'Darling, you can't sign anymore. That method has gone out. You now have to put a PIN number in my machine here!' - pointing towards her machine.

'I do not use Chip and PIN! I sign for payments!'

'We don't do that anymore. Give me your card and tell me your number and I'll do it all for you.'

'I will not give you my number; I want to sign.'

'But you can't do that any more. If you won't give me your PIN, give it to your carer. She can do it for you!'

Taking hold of Kathleen's arm, I retaliated, 'This is my wife, not my carer, and I'm getting rather angry. The law says I do not have to use Chip and PIN; I can sign. I will not give my PIN to anyone. So please get on with it and let me sign!'

By this time, quite a queue had formed behind me and the assistant addressed them: 'I'm sorry for the delay. He doesn't understand. I don't think he can help it!'

I had to restrain Kathleen and requested that she keep quiet.

My anger was obvious as I shouted very loudly, 'I understand perfectly. It is you who don't understand. Get me the manager now!'

She tried to say something but, leaning over the counter and putting my face as close to hers as I could, I shouted in my anger, 'Get the manager - now!'

So loud was my voice that the assistant didn't need to call the manager; he appeared and asked, 'Is there something wrong?'

Giving him a venomous look, I informed him, 'Yes, there is something wrong. This apology for a human being is humiliating me and making me feel like a complete idiot. Are you and the staff trained in disability awareness and the Disability Discrimination Act?'

He cautiously replied, 'Yes. We've all had training!'

Looking straight into his eyes, I retorted, 'The people in the queue behind me are all witnesses to the treatment I've received here today. I want to pay for our shopping using my credit card. I don't want to use Chip and PIN; I want to sign for them!'

'That's no problem, sir,' he replied, bobbing down and producing the relevant machine and form for me to sign.

It took seconds to solve my problem.

The assistant spoke to the manager in surprised tones, 'I didn't know that was there. I didn't know we could still use that!'

The manager gave her a look which conveyed the message 'I'll deal with you later'.

He then gathered up our bags of shopping and offered them to me in a dismissive way. I did not take the shopping. I stood and made it obvious by the look on my face and my body language that our business was not complete.

'Is there something more?' He questioned.

'I think there is,' said I, 'I am actually waiting for an apology!'

'I am so sorry,' offered the manager!

'You're sorry!?' I retorted. 'I think the apology should come from your assistant, don't you?'

The offending assistant had moved along the counter to another till and was serving another customer. Without looking up from her work, she called to me from a distance, 'I'm sorry darling! But you're alright now. All's well that ends well!'

The manager smiled at me as much as to say, 'there you are, you've got your apology; you can go now'.

I was far from happy and all was not well. However, my anger was controlled but evident. I was also aware of the queue that had formed behind me. I felt I had to assert myself and redeem my self-respect.

'That was the most insincere apology I've ever heard. I will not leave this store until I get a proper apology. An apology offered face-to-face!'

Someone in the queue behind me shouted 'Hear, hear!' and I was encouraged by that. Eventually, the assistant came over to me and spoke with disdain, 'I have apologised. What more do you want – blood?'

'I'm afraid so! I want you to look me in the eye and apologise. But I want you to know what you are apologising for. I want you to know how you made me feel. This is not all about me. It's also about people who come after me!'

Looking a little lost for words and also rather embarrassed, the woman replied, 'I don't know what you want me to say. I've already said I'm sorry!'

'You said you were sorry from a distance. It was not acceptable to me. It was not meant –it was insincere!'

'Well, I'm sorry. I didn't know you could still sign I thought it was all Chip and PIN now!'

'This is not about your lack of knowledge. It's about your attitude. It's about how you made me feel. When I was tying my shoe lace earlier, you made comments to my wife. How rude was that? I can tie my shoe any way I want. I don't comment on the way you tie your laces. Then you assume and say my wife is my carer and question it by the look on your face when I put you right. I wonder, were you questioning my manhood or were you thinking no one could marry something like that? And then you announced to the entire shop that I don't understand and you don't think I can help it, thereby bringing my mental faculties into question. Not only embarrassing me and making me feel an idiot but doing it in front of my wife! I think you were wondering why I need an apology - maybe now you understand!'

There was at this point applause from some of the people in the queue behind us, who had obviously witnessed some of the treatment I had received.

The manager intervened and suggested 'we take it into the office' but my humiliation had been in public. I wanted an apology in public.

The woman was almost in tears and I did feel sorry for her but I was thinking of other people who might not have had the confidence I had or even the language I had. I don't usually challenge people so aggressively or determinedly but this woman put my back up. Her attitude and her aura were offensive to me.

Eventually, I did receive an apology. But that wasn't good enough for me and I continued to badger until the woman apologised again and confessed that she had learned from the experience and would be more careful in what she said to people in the future.

Kathleen is usually very placid. She speaks her mind and we do have differences of opinions but we do not quarrel much. But on this occasion, when we returned to the car, she had things to say:

'You were a bit rough on that woman! Was it really necessary? It could all have been avoided. I could have put your PIN in for you!'

'Kathleen, you know as well as I do, it's the principal of the thing.'

'I don't agree. You took a dislike to the woman and you let her have it and I think you were out of order. What impression did you give to that woman of disabled people? You reacted like a crip with a chip! How do you think she is going to react to other disabled people after your onslaught? I think it was all very unnecessary. It's not like you're going to meet that woman ever again. She isn't going to be a permanent part of our lives!'

As always, Kathleen provided food for thought. She did make me wonder why I could take an instant dislike to a person I didn't know and why I allowed such people to bring out the worse in me. Kathleen commented that I usually use humour in these situations and still get my point across.

Will I ever learn!? And why, oh why is Kathleen always right!?

***

As a trainer, I met all kinds of people and whilst making a training film for a national bank I met a man with cerebral palsy. He was affected by this

183

similarly to me. The only difference was that he needed a translator to repeat the words he spoke!

We became very good friends because we had so much in common. Not only did we share the same experience of cerebral palsy, we also shared a similar sense of humour. We were wicked together! People named us the terrible twins.

I involved him in some of my training courses as a co-trainer. He was reluctant to do this at first because of his speech but after the first course he gained confidence and enthusiasm.

We were both invited to a posh do in the House of Lords through meeting people as I worked for central government departments. We were both excited by the invitation and decided that we should look around for trendy evening wear. We were aware that we could hire a conventional diner jacket outfit but we wanted to be modern and trendy.

Our homes were in different towns and he didn't drive so we arranged to meet in a large city centre shopping complex nearer to his home than mine.

As we looked around the various menswear shops, we noticed that velvet brocade jackets were the in thing. We went into a well-known high street store and began trying on these lovely jackets. I must say here that although he had his translator with him, I didn't need her, for I was well tuned in to his speech as he was to mine. So as we were trying on jackets, we were talking, joking with each other and laughing. Our behaviour accentuated the effects of our cerebral palsy!

I had chosen a maroon-coloured jacket and he had chosen a blue. I approached an assistant, who was adequately proportioned and looked rather matronly, and asked where trousers were. She replied, quite haughtily I thought:

'These are rather expensive and very modern. There are some cheaper and more traditional evening suits down there!' and she indicated the back of the shop.

It wasn't just what she said but the way she said it along with her body language and facial expression.

Before I could retaliate, my friend, using his translator, said, 'We'll leave the jackets for now. I'd like to look at ties.' With this, he handed the two jackets to the woman assistant to put back on their hangers.

By this time in our friendship, I knew him well and the look in his eyes and on his face told me he was up to something. And through his translator, he said to the assistant:

'Can you show us the ties, please?'

The assistant took us to the ties and my friend said again through his translator.

'Me and my mate here have great problems controlling our dribble so we are looking for dribble-proof ties. We are both public speakers and it looks awful when we dribble down our ties when we are in public!'

I could feel giggles and laughter welling up from the depth of me. I was also amazed at the serious face on the translator as she repeated my friend's words to the shop assistant. I was also impressed by the shop assistant, who seemed to understand the problem, for she answered. 'I have the solution right here,' indicating a selection of ties!

'These are Teflon-coated and could be just what you're looking for!'

'Oh no!' replied my friend! 'They are no good! With Teflon-coated, the dribble runs off on to our trousers and it looks like we have peed ourselves!'

I had to run from the shop because the giggles and the laughter that I had hitherto controlled erupted! I had to drop onto a seat until my spasm of giggles subsided.

It wasn't only what was said but the way my friend's translator said it with a pan face that didn't express any mirth or humour.

I don't know what was said in the shop after I left but as we three all met afterwards, we were unable to speak to one another. We hung on to each other's' shoulders in a bunch and we shook with laughter for some considerable time!

We found another shop which sold the same jackets but knowing how we would react if we went in the shop together, I sent him in first. He purchased his blue velvet jacket and left the shop and I entered the shop to buy mine. But there was no maroon one on the rack so I went to the till to inquire if they might have one in the back of the shop. The assistant on the till told me he had sold the last maroon one not ten minutes ago. I had to leave the shop rather hastily because my friend was looking through the shop window, which was behind the till, pulling faces at me, making hand gestures and miming tying a tie and I had no control left!

When I met up with him outside the shop, I had to take a deep breath and I said, 'Now look! We are both behaving quite juvenile. Let's calm down!'

He looked at me with a serious face and said to no one in particular:

'He's grumpy because they hadn't got the jacket he wanted and he's jealous because I've got mine.'

'You stay there and wait for me. I'll go back to the other shop and buy the one I tried on earlier.'

'No you won't!'

'I beg your pardon!? What do you mean - no I won't?'

'I mean you won't go back to that other shop because I've got the maroon one. When I bought mine, I could see they only had one in maroon and other people were looking at them, so I bought it for you. It is the size you wanted.'

'You let me go in that shop knowing they hadn't got what I wanted and knowing you'd bought one for me. I could have bought another colour, a green one or a black one.'

'No, I wouldn't have let you buy another one. I was watching you through the window. Good fun here, isn't it?'

***

The demand for training courses in personal development increased and I continued to learn so much about myself through facilitating these courses. I learned I had attitudes and prejudices which affected my behaviour and I learned how I needed to analyse my attitudes and prejudices in order to form better and more meaningful relationships in both my business life and my social life. I also learned that most of my attitudes could not be got rid of but because I was aware of them, I tried to ensure that they no longer affected my behaviour. Surprisingly, I discovered most of my attitudes and prejudices were formed in my childhood through early experiences and family and community influences. It was also interesting to learn by really analysing my feelings that many of my attitudes and prejudices were linked to my habits, and the habits of a lifetime are really difficult to erase. Those habits caused me to ignore certain individuals and groups of people and it soon became obvious that I was missing out on many experiences and on learning and sharing through habits formed by my attitudes and prejudices! It took time to change but then I discovered the great value in sharing talents and in the intermingling of culture and I realised, to my regret, that maybe I had missed out on business opportunities because, opposed to popular belief, disabled people are not all white. I was able to extend what courses I offered by researching the issues for disabled people whose culture, skin colour and background were different and facilitated quite a few courses in this area.

I wasn't very comfortable working with other cultures. After all, I had issues with non-disabled people facilitating training in disability issues. I was aware that these non-disabled trainers did a good job, got the message across and were allies to the cause but they lacked the real personal experience of living with a disability. Likewise, I lacked the experience of living with cultural differences. So I trained two people, one with an Asian background and one with an Afro-Caribbean background; both had disability and both had difficulty getting a job. I kept them in work for about eight months and they both became self-employed. I was disappointed because we lost touch after a short while but I excused them because I know how demanding running one's own business can be!

As I progressed and met more people, I also learned of the many issues facing disabled people working for central government departments, and so I was able to give advice on training needs for non-disabled people working in these departments. I was hoping that my advice and recommendations would bring in more work with non-disabled people but there was minimal response!

It was on a personal development course that I met Sandra. She was thirty-one years of age and had worked for the department as a clerical assistant for the last eight years. I first met her in the hotel reception area.

Her face was void of any expression and she had a drooping eyelid. It was as though she were wearing a blank mask. I must confess I was a bit shocked! Her complexion was flawless but stark white and alabaster-looking. Her appearance did not convey self-confidence. Her deportment was 'slumped' and she didn't look up; her gaze was always down on the ground.

I had encountered people with facial disfigurements before and I wasn't very good with them. Where did one look when speaking to a person with a facial disfigurement? Social rules demanded that one looked at the face when speaking to another person! I wasn't very comfortable looking into Sandra's face as I spoke to her; I felt like I was staring at her or maybe felt that Sandra might think I was staring at her. I did wish someone had warned me! But then again, I would hate others to warn people of me! Once again, I had to recognise my attitudes and face my fears and by doing this, I learned of myself and developed from doing so.

Although the department sent notes on each student prior to a personal development course, I did not read much. I was interested in people's needs. I needed to know how best to facilitate them in the training room and in the domestic areas but I liked to get to know people rather than be influenced by others' comments. I was aware that I had been prejudiced in the past by reading pre-course notes. I did not understand medical labels anyway and I also knew from personal and past experience that people were very individual and each person's experience and manifestation, even of the same medical label, was vastly different.

Maybe to compensate for my awful attitudes or maybe to hide my awful attitudes towards Sandra's lack of facial expression, I gave her a little more attention than the others. Actually, it soon became obvious that Sandra needed that attention! She wasn't freely forthcoming in training sessions. If she could, she would sit in the back corner of the training room and remain quiet! I really had to ask her direct questions in order to involve her. She would never volunteer any answers or information. It was difficult for me, for not being able to read any facial expressions whatsoever, I wasn't sure that my attention was putting her under undue pressure.

It was at Sandra's personal tutorial that she explained her situation to me.

Two years earlier she had been diagnosed with myasthenia gravis. Sandra explained that she had weakness of muscles, particularly to her face. She did not have any pain. Sandra said sometimes she had difficulty in chewing and swallowing. She said she got very tired towards the end of the day.

Apparently, myasthenia gravis is caused by abnormal antibodies in the bloodstream that the immune system cannot deal with. These antibodies upset the workings of chemicals, which help the nerves convey messages to the muscles! The production of these abnormal antibodies can sometimes be associated with the thymos gland in the chest. This gland has an active part in the immune system.

Sandra had been told that her thymos gland appeared to be healthy and because of this, Sandra was really confused as to what had caused her to have the disease. It was obvious that Sandra was being cared for by her medical professionals, as she reported a wide variety of therapies which had been tried. She had had blood transfusions too, which removed antibodies from the blood and the transfusions had had a good effect but had not been very long-lasting.

Sandra had been told by her doctors that she would regain near-normal function of her muscles in time as research into therapies and treatments progressed!

A personal tutorial gave each student the opportunity to talk about personal issues that may have arisen from the content of the course or may not have been covered by the course. It was also hoped that students would be helped to formulate their action plans to aid their future development. It was also an opportunity to research sources of help and information according to each individual's needs.

My usual opening to a personal tutorial was to ask the student how they had found the course and to follow that by asking them to tell me the most important thing they had learned from the course.

Sandra did not really respond to my general questions; she seemed to have her own agenda for her tutorial and I welcomed this but was not prepared for the questions and issues raised.

'Alan!' began Sandra, 'You have unusual facial movements and grimaces. How do you cope?'

I really was thrown by her question. I knew I had a muscle spasm that caused twitches and the effort of speaking often made my face contort.

'Sandra, I really don't know what to say. Talk to me more about your question and hopefully I'll be able to respond meaningfully!'

'Well, the biggest issue for me is people staring at me. They stare at my face and it really gets to me and I thought you must experience the same problems because of your facial movements.'

'Sandra, I'm sure people do stare at me but most of the time I am able to ignore them. Usually, I'm too busy to be self-conscious. I always have something to think about, which helps me not to be aware of others staring at me!'

'How can you ignore people who stare at you?'

'Well, I've had a life time of practice. I'm a lot older than you, so I've had a lot of time to work things out. But I must admit I do get annoyed with parents who say to their kids, it's rude to stare or it's rude to ask questions. If kids want to know about me, I'll tell them. All they need are simple explanations and they're happy. I think parents make things worse, they make disability a mystery or a no-no, and they are just as curious as their children! So you see, I don't like ignoring the younger generation, providing they're not rude!'

'That's so interesting. I've learned such a lot this week and from my tutorial I was hoping to learn how to cope better with people who stare.'

'Sandra, for me it's how I cope with my own self consciousness rather than coping with people who stare at me.'

This was one of the most difficult tutorials I had ever conducted because I was not receiving any non-verbal feedback or clues as to how Sandra was receiving what I was saying because of the total lack of any facial expression.

I had found a way of coping with my difficulties in looking at Sandra. I looked at her forehead or her chin or her ears. I avoided making eye contact – that was really too uncomfortable for me. I hoped that this was acceptable to Sandra.

'Do you know, Alan, I've never thought of it like that before. What you are saying is I need to cope with my feelings, rather than concern myself with what others might be thinking when they stare at me!'

'Something like that, but we'll look at the situation in a different way, have we? Imagine - You come out of your home one morning and there's an ambulance parked down the road with the back doors open and the blue lights still flashing. What would you do?'

'I'd be commenting to my husband. I'd want to know what's going on!'

'Why Sandra, why would you want to know what's going on?'

'Well, maybe because of my curiosity!'

'Could it be, that just maybe, because you're a nosey bugger, Sandra?' I said with a smile on my face and a twinkle in my eye. I knew that Sandra couldn't laugh or smile at my comment but she grabbed my forearm to show she accepted my comment as humour.

'Okay, Sandra! Imagine - you're in a bus queue and in front of you there is a young man with a bandage round his head, a real shiner of a black eye and his arm in a sling. What would you do? Would you stare at him and look away if he looked at you?'

'I would, wouldn't I? I'd stare at him. I'd be curious, wouldn't I?'

'So Sandra, why do people stare at you?'

'Could it be because they're curious, just like I am with others?'

'Sandra, when you stare at people, do you have thoughts which condemn them because of their appearance or do you have kinder thoughts? Do you have sympathy?'

'You are really making me think now, Alan. I think if it was a young man with black eyes and such, I might think he'd been in a drunken brawl and I might condemn. But anything else, I think I'd feel sympathetic.'

'What are you thinking now, Sandra?'

'I can't put it into words. I need time to sort it out in my head.'

'There are other things I want to discuss with you but do you want me to go on or do you want a break and we'll talk again tomorrow?'

190

'I really want to carry on. There are some other people in the office I work in who say you made them see things differently and they are better for it. So I want to carry on.'

'Now Sandra, I want you to be really honest with me. I am not easily offended and you can't embarrass me. So be honest!'

Normally people would react to this statement and that reaction might show in the person's facial expression and I might judge their feelings through their facial expressions. With Sandra, I heard what she said but I could not judge the full meaning of her words because of the lack of even the slightest movement in her face. I found this really difficult.

I shifted in my seat to a more comfortable position (or maybe to cover up my discomfort) and I offered:

'I'm going to carry on, but tell me if you want to stop or need a break. Tell me if you become distressed.'

Sandra adjusted her sitting position in her chair as though bracing herself for what was to follow.

'Tell me, Sandra, what did you think of me the first time you met me? Remember when you arrived at the hotel on the first day of the course. I met you in the foyer and said hello. What did you think?'

'I can't tell you that!'

'Yes you can, Sandra. I really want you to tell me!'

There was hesitation and a reticence and I helped her out by injecting:

'Sandra, did you think, "He can't be our trainer! I must not have heard him right. I'm sure he said I'm your trainer! How's he going to run a training course?" Along with, "I can't understand his speech." And I bet you thought, "I want to go home now". You also wondered who in the department gave me the job as trainer! Am I right?'

There was a silence and Sandra fidgeted on her chair and I could tell she did not want to answer.

'Oh come on, Sandra. You thought all of this and more. Didn't you? Just tell me.'

'This is embarrassing, Alan!'

'Embarrassing? Embarrassing to who: you or me?'

Again, I felt she was reluctant to answer and I had to encourage:

'I'm right, aren't I? And you are not alone. The others in the group had similar thoughts! I know, Sandra! I've been around a long time!'

She nodded her head and so I continued:

'You've changed your mind, haven't you? Your initial thoughts of me have changed. Why?'

I could tell by the atmosphere between us that she wasn't going to answer but I'm sure she was thinking.

'Sandra. Are you okay? This is really difficult. What I've said so far may have sounded aggressive and sarcastic. It's all said to make you think.'

'You are making me think and you are right. I've changed my initial thoughts about you!'

'Sandra. What I'm going to say now is said to make you think. I'm not criticising and I'm not trying to hurt.'

'Well, you have given me lots to think about already.'

'Sandra. I want to ask you three questions. I don't want you to answer them. I want you to go away and think about them. 1st question: if I had hidden away in a corner and not spoken, would that have reinforced the negatives you already thought? 2nd question: if I had sat separately in the dinning room, what would you have thought? 3rd question: does the change in your thinking towards me have anything to do with my behaviour?'

There was silence in the room and suddenly she rendered, 'I must look a real fool! Thank you for saying those things!'

'Hey, don't thank me, please. I have more to say. I feel I'm being hard on you and I really don't want to upset you. Believe me, Sandra, I know how difficult it is for you.'

'I think it's relatively easy for me because if I am aware someone is staring at me, I can smile at them and maybe through my facial expression let them know I'm happy being me. Sometimes I have been known to say to people who stare, "I was born like this and I'm used to it. I'm happy being me." I think people also react to confidence and I can convey that through body language and posture. Does that make any sense to you?'

'Yes, Alan, it does. I'm going to have to change, aren't I? I'm now thinking I'm my own worst enemy!'

'No; don't even think that! What's happened to you is really difficult to get used to. I think you have done well. You've carried on working – that must have been terribly hard for you. I assume you are married because you're wearing a wedding ring. (She nodded.) That must be a tender area! And to come away on a residential course like this – wow, that took guts. So I admire you. I think you are doing really well!'

'Thank you, Alan. It really helps to talk with someone who understands.'

'Sandra. My issues might be different to yours. Firstly, I'm a man and I think there are gender issues involved – maybe in all disabilities! We may share similar experiences inasmuch as people look at me and assume my intelligence or ability is limited or I'm shy or have no confidence and people think I have not or will not achieve anything. Many people assume my wife is my carer and that, more than anything else, makes me angry. How dare people question my manhood! I've even been asked by many if my children are adopted!'

'Oh Alan, how do you cope? How do I cope?'

'Sandra, I cope the best way I can. I reckon I have a right to be happy and I'm not going to allow others to take away that right. I also have a network of friends who put me back together should I fall apart and the most important thing for me is my wife and family. I have a big responsibility towards them and that really motivates me.'

'From now on I'm going to change, Alan. The first thing I'm going to do is phone my husband and put things right with him. I've been a devil to him. I've taken all my frustrations out on him. From now on I'm not going to hide away in corners or even sit on the back row! I'm going to sit on the front row and have my say!'

'Good for you, Sandra! But you make it sound easy and it's not. Just remember the face is how you communicate; it tells people who we are and when we look in a mirror the face is our self-image. You and I are the same as other people inasmuch as we are obsessed with our looks, our appearance, with our own self-image! I'm afraid you and I break all the norms of acceptability and we have got to come to terms with who we are and what we are before we can tackle the big wide world.'

'Alan, you have made it very clear that I have a big battle on my hands but I now know my enemy. It's not the big wide world. It's me and I tell you I'm going to change!'

'Now, I want to add a word of caution here! I am speaking from my own personal experience! In trying to change, you might put yourself under enormous stress and you may fail and that will cause even more stress, so think about that change very carefully and define small achievable steps. With a medical condition, stress can make things worse, so watch it.'

'You are very wise, Alan. I feel like I'm talking to someone who knows – someone who has been there and done that.'

'Yep! I don't change myself or my behaviour without analysing why, now! If change will benefit me financially, health-wise or work-wise or if it will improve any relationships, especially with my wife or family, I'll try it. But I will not change to fit in with the crowd or to become more acceptable to a particular person. I had to learn to accept myself and like myself as I am. I'm constantly trying to improve things in my life – I want to be kinder and become more sensitive to the needs of my wife and family but there are things I cannot change. Sometimes I'm quiet and sit on the back row and I reckon that's okay. It can take effort to sit on the front row and open my mouth and I have to assess: is it worth the effort? Basically I'm shy and lacking in confidence and I really have to push myself to be otherwise. But I don't need to push myself all the time. It's okay for me to take a back seat sometimes. Change can be stressful and I really had to learn how to manage stress; it can have a detrimental effect on my functioning. I have to manage stress or it might manage me. I really have to be aware of what I'm doing and why I'm doing it! I'm looking for fulfilment and value in life and in my work and that should not be too stressful!'

Sandra took hold of my arm and I didn't really know what that meant to convey, but after a brief moment of silence she spoke:

'Do you know, Alan, many people tell me what I should do, including my husband. Sometimes I feel like I'm being preached at. But you have not told me what I should or should not do. You have shared your personal experiences and that's really helped and made me think. You have given me such a lot to think about. I want to go now and phone my husband but I assure you I will not hold my head in shame anymore. I'm going to take far more care of myself after this!'

'Sandra. I hope you're happy with your time in this tutorial. I feel like I've talked too much. I usually get the student to talk to me!' at this point she interrupted.

'It's what I needed!'

We ended our meeting with a hug, and Sandra went off to phone her husband. She arrived at dinner, sat with the rest of the group and chatted to other students for the first time during the course.

The following morning, Sandra sat on the front row of the training room and contributed without any encouragement.

After our morning refreshment break, I had time to ask Sandra how things

194

were going for her after her tutorial and she replied, 'Amazingly! I made the first move at dinner last evening and now every one is speaking to me. A lot of it is up to me isn't it?'

'I'm afraid so, Sandra. It is easier here on the course because we are all in the same boat. Back at the office you may be very alone.'

'But before I became ill those people at the office were my friends and I've ostracised myself. I'm sure I can repair the damage!'

'Good luck to you, Sandra.' I had to curtail our conversation with Sandra to resume training.

***

Kathleen and I often look back to the course Sandra attended and we refer to it as 'that was the course that was'. We had a young man with epilepsy and he had three and four fits a day. This was very distracting for the group as well as hard work for me. So disruptive too! On the third morning he appeared in the training room; he looked dreadful and confessed to me that he felt terribly ill. I asked if he could be exhausted because of all the fits he had had that week. He agreed with me so I sent him back to bed to have a long sleep.

A woman from the hotel office called me out of the training room mid-morning and told me that one of the hotel's domestic staff had found one of my students dead on the floor of his bedroom. The hotel had called the police and the ambulance.

Sure enough, it was our student with epilepsy!

I dashed to his bedroom and as he lay on the floor he was surrounded by women; I think all were domestic staff.

After an epileptic seizure, he went into a very deep sleep and I knew that what I was seeing was the aftereffect of a fit. I pinched his ears and his cheeks and this aroused him. I shook him until he was fully awake and as he arose from the floor all the women screamed and ran from the room. I think they thought I had raised the dead!

The ambulance and the police were cancelled but I had had enough. I was commissioned as a trainer, not a nurse or a carer, so I called his line manager, who was very surprised that he was on the course as he had been on sick leave for the past month because of his frequent fits and as he hadn't produced a final medical certificate, he was not expected to attend the course.

I must admit I responded to this information a little aggressively and someone arranged for the British Red Cross to come to the hotel and transport him home!

***

Also during the course, Kathleen and I had been woken early one morning, about 2 a.m., by the police, who had arrested one of our students for brawling and fighting outside a public house in the nearby town. Another male student was also involved and I had no other option but to send them home. The government department had a code of behaviour for residential courses and brawling outside a public house violated this code! Unfortunately, my action in sending these men home was not approved of by their line managers but I saw it as beyond my call of duty to have to deal with louts.

Luckily, my decision was upheld by the manager of my contract but it was still not a nice situation to have to deal with.

***

It was my practice to begin a training course by having everyone introduce themselves. This was to enable me to learn the name of each student. One of the male students had a problem telling me his name, which concerned me somewhat. On questioning him it became clear that his confusion was because at home he was called one name by his parents and another name by his work colleagues. He could not decide which name to use on the course and the other delegates decided for him.

This forty-year-old man found it difficult to make any decisions. I discovered him at 7:30 on the first morning of the course in dressing gown and slippers, in reception phoning 'mummy' and asking her what to wear and what he should have for breakfast!

I had a personal interview with him before I began training that day and after quite a lengthy discussion, he agreed that he would decide what to wear and what to eat without phoning mum. He did confess that he had to phone mummy each morning and each evening to tell her that he had remembered to take his medication. This was for epilepsy. He hadn't had a fit for many years.

I had a dilemma! Did my role as trainer give me the right to request that this 40-year-old man take control of his own life, make decisions for himself and stop calling his mum 'mummy'? I'm afraid it was the way he said 'mummy' which grated on me rather than the actual word. I need not have worried because something happened on the first day of training. Whether it was the content of the programme or comments from other students or a combination of both, I'll never know, but at the end of that first day he came to me and timidly asked, 'I'm going to phone mum and tell her I won't forget to take my tablets and I won't phone her again this week. Do you think that would be the right thing to do?'

My reply was, 'I can't tell you what to do. You decide for yourself!'

Apparently, he did phone mum!

On the last night of the course we were all invited to the local pub for karaoke. I was concerned that there might be flashing lights, which might trigger epilepsy for our student. He assured me he was not affected by flashing lights but maybe he should not go as mum didn't allow him to go in pubs.

I was aware of a discussion among the students at the meal table. The prevalent comment I heard was, 'Look, you're miles away from home. How's your mum going to know you've been in a pub? It's time you enjoyed yourself. What your mum doesn't know won't hurt her!'

He was there at the karaoke!

One of the men sitting very near to us was obviously celebrating his birthday and his friends had ordered a strip-a-gram for him.

Our student dashed to watch the proceedings with protruding eyes and then announced to the assembled group:

'Flashing lights don't affect my epilepsy but flashing boobs might!'

***

One young man on the same course was said to have learning difficulties. He had a great deal to contribute to the course in each discussion and training session and he was very popular with the other students. He seemed to be sensitive and caring and if he saw someone had a need, he would offer help.

I was impressed by him. He worked in the Queen's Warehouse. That's where illegal goods confiscated by police and custom officers are stored until the importing agent, individual or gang have been dealt with by the courts and then the illegal goods are destroyed or sent to an incinerator and burned.

I would say our student could not read or write and I questioned if, in fact, he had learning difficulties. His social skills were good and his linguistic contributions to the course demonstrated his intellect and his speed of thinking.

His line manager seemed to be very caring and was looking to 'promote' this young man from menial duties to something with a little responsibility.

Since our young student had a driving licence and indeed drove his own car, I suggested he was coached and ultimately took the department's driving test with a view to him driving goods from the warehouse to the incinerator.

In due course, I received news that our starred student had passed the departmental driving test and was now an official driver for the Queen's Warehouse!

Whether the additional news was true I cannot say – it reported that he had loaded confiscated cigarettes into his van and had secured the rear door but left one of the side doors open. So as he drove from the warehouse to the incinerator, he left a trail of cigarettes on the road behind him! If this is true, all I can say is, we all make mistakes. Hopefully we learn from them.

I have heard that our young man is very popular with the general public who live on the route from the warehouse to the incinerator!!!

***

Sandra and I kept in touch. She emailed me every week. She did well on her return to the office. Apparently she spoke about the effects of myasthenia gravis, which she experienced at a team meeting at the office and this was received with interest and compassion. Sandra confessed that telling the team about her problems was the hardest thing she ever did but it had paid enormous dividends! Her former friendships with members of the office team had resumed and she had more support from the team. Sandra was happier in her work and I suggest when we are happy, we are less stressed and we are more able to cope with our problems.

Sandra was also happier in her marriage. She carried out my suggestion that she spoke with her husband about how Sandra's condition affected him. This she did and through this discussion they understood each other better and their communication improved.

Many times, people who acquire a disability become quite insular, if not selfish. I think that's understandable but any disability doesn't just affect the individual, it affects the whole family. I know from experience that the individual gets all the attention from the medical profession and other services and more often than not gets much support, care and comfort from family but often the issues of other family members caused by disability are completely ignored!

It was some months after the course that I was working quite near to Sandra's home and she invited me to dinner to meet her husband. Meeting strangers for social occasions is not my favourite thing to do and on occasions

I can be quite innovative in creating excuses, but because it was Sandra, I felt I had to accept her invitation.

For our meeting she had chosen a new restaurant that had opened on the outskirts of town. On enquiring about this new eating place, I was told it was a bit 'swanky'. The building had been built many years ago as a convent and had always been home to an order of nuns. Now it had been transformed into a rather expensive residential five star hotel!

I arrived early to enable me to look around because I was interested in the history of the building and I thought I might use some of the information I gained as conversational pieces during dinner.

The reception area of the hotel was lavishly but tastefully decorated. The pile on the maroon and blue carpet was so thick, it almost covered one's shoe as you entered the hotel. The staff in the reception area wore uniform of maroon with blue lapels and stripes up the side seams of their trousers or skirts and there was a welcoming atmosphere.

There wasn't information on the history of the building displayed in the reception area and whilst looking around, I was approached by a member of staff who asked if I needed help. I explained that I was meeting friends for dinner and while I was waiting, I was looking for information on the history of the building. The man asked me to wait and left me standing in the reception area and returned with a female who was not wearing uniform but was the deputy manager of the hotel. (This I gleaned from the name badge she wore on the label badge of the jacket she wore.)

I told her that I had heard of the previous use of the building and I was interested in the original architecture and the process of renovation to the present and thought there might be something displayed as I felt more people than I may have had the same interest.

The deputy manager explained that there had been long debates by the hotel's management team on displaying the information I was looking for but all they could offer me was an album of photographs and press cuttings of before and after.

I found the album really interesting and it promoted conversation between us. Sometimes one can meet a stranger and have an instant rapport with them and that how it was with us. I felt the deputy manager was a person I could get on with.

As we proceeded to look through the photographs, I commented on all kinds of structural issues. Whilst I was really interested in the building and in particular, the renovations, I could not help commenting on aspects of disability. Because of the narrowness of doors on the old plans, I questioned if one could pursue a strong vocation and become a nun if one was a wheelchair user. I questioned the small confessional box and I talked about the issues of a blind nun who needed a guide dog! The convent chapel had steps going down to it and whilst the photographs depicted the splendour of the chapel area with a very ornate altar, once again I was aware of how difficult it might be for women with various disabilities to follow a vocation as a nun!

The deputy manager seemed to be interested in all the issues I raised and then we discussed the renovation and the present architectural structure of the hotel. I asked about wheelchair access because I didn't see a ramp by the entrance and I was not at all sure a wheelchair would get through the revolving door which I had used to enter the building. I doubted if I could have got through the revolving door had I had luggage! So I assumed a person using crutches or having a guide dog would have difficulties with the restrictions imposed by the revolving doors. I was supposed to be assured by the assistant manager's comments:

'No problems there. We always have a man on the door to deal with luggage. It would be taken from our guests and brought into the hotel through a side door and delivered to the relevant bedroom or suite.'

I was interested to hear more about the use of the side door and so I asked, 'What about wheel chairs and guide dogs and such things?'

'Again, they would be brought through the side door and straight up to their rooms. We also offer a free room service to anyone with a disability.'

'Well, that's really interesting. My friends will be arriving soon and I don't think we have time to discuss all the issues that your comments raise. Let me give you my business card. Do you get many disabled people staying here?'

'No we don't. We have been open just ten months and I think we've had one person in a wheelchair and one blind woman.'

'Wow. I think you are missing out on a lot of business. It is estimated by the Office for National Statistics that there are at least 6,000,000 disabled people in the UK (this estimate relates to the 1990s). I consider that to be a low estimate but if I were in a business like yours, I'd like to attract that large portion of our society. Not only attract disabled people but they would bring their family and friends with them too! Think of all those people and all the cash they could bring to your business!'

'That's amazing!' commented the woman, 'I'd never thought of disability in terms of a business issue!'

I could see that Sandra and her husband were entering the reception area and were walking towards us so I had to curtail my conversation with the deputy manager but I reminded her that she had my business card and my contact details.

It was good to see Sandra walking through reception on the arm of her husband. She carried herself erect. Gone were the slouching shoulders of the past. Her eyes were not downcast as on the course but she looked interested in her surroundings and this in itself created a certain confidence in her appearance. There was also a smile in her eyes too, which I had noticed had developed since I last saw her on the course. She still had no expression whatsoever – she had not recovered any tone in her facial muscles – but she had lost the forlorn and weary look.

Sandra introduced me to Rob, her husband, who was a really well-built man with rippling muscles and large hands, which indicated to me that he was a manual worker, for they were ingrained with dirt.

We shook hands and exchanged niceties and followed the deputy manager's directions to the hotel's restaurant.

The deco in the restaurant was spectacular. It was a very large ground floor room. The walls were painted grey but the type of paint used made the walls appear as though they were covered in satin. Large pictures hung on the walls, each one in an elaborately ornate gold-coloured frame depicting restful rural scenes which, I was told, were scenes of actual sights surrounding the town. The ceiling was also very decorative - fancy plaster work in a floral pattern, with the flowers painted in various pastel colours, with gold-coloured garlands of leaves entwined within the flowers. The carpet was a plain maroon colour and the tables were covered with pale blue linen cloths. Each dining chair had a little gold-coloured scrolling on the back.

As we entered the room, the maître d' met us and spoke directly to Rob.

'Good Evening sir – do you have a booking?'

'Yes, we have a booking,' replied Sandra, 'I booked by phone a few days ago.'

The maître d' absolutely ignored Sandra and again looked directly at Rob as he responded, 'Just a moment and I'll find you on our booking plan.'

Unfortunately for some people, I had learned to lip-read whilst working in the cotton mill and it's a skill that I have retained, so when the maître d' approached the younger woman behind the desk, I could read what the woman was saying. Apparently we had been allocated one table at the time of booking but now, for some obscure reason, that initial allocation would need to be changed and we were assigned to another table.

My very suspicious mind began to work and I wondered why our table had to be changed. Had they double-booked or was there some other reason? I did not see the woman say anything to the maître d' about the table being double booked!

We were escorted by the maître d' to a table in the far corner of the room and I felt we were being hidden away. My suspicions were reinforced as I looked around and noticed the tables around the centre of the room were reserved but the tables where we had been placed did not have reserved notices on them!

I didn't want to upset Sandra or Rob. So I excused myself and quietly asked if I could speak with the maître d' away from my friends. He was so polite and condescending as I walked with him a little way down the restaurant. Out of earshot of Sandra, I assertively challenged:

'I don't like the table you have assigned to us. Could you change it, please?'

'I'm afraid not,' he lied, 'That's the only table available - all the others are booked, sir!'

'I am sorry but I know that's not true. You see, I can lip-read and I know what that woman behind the desk said to you! When my friend booked our meal by telephone she was allocated a specific table. Now when she is seen to have a facial disfigurement or maybe you become aware of my disability, I suspect, our allocated table is changed to one in the corner where we cannot be seen. Apart from that, most of the tables in the centre of the room have reserved notices on them but the tables around where we have been seated don't have any reserved notices on them. I feel you are trying to hide us away!'

His denial and the fact that he avoided making eye contact with me aggravated me further and, rather than lose my temper, I asked to see the deputy manager. After a brief telephone call made by the woman behind the desk, I was told that the deputy manager was not available.

'Really!?' I replied. 'We will see about that!' As I walked to exit the restaurant, I exclaimed over my shoulder, 'I'll be back shortly.'

I went to the main reception desk and gave my name and asked if I could see the deputy manager. Of course, the receptionist wanted to know why I wanted to see the deputy manager and looking directly into his eyes, I addressed the receptionist with directness:

'Young man, up until now I have been cool, calm and collected. But if you don't want a scene on your hands, I should call the deputy manager now. Look, there are many people milling around and I don't mind letting them know of the awful treatment I have received in this hotel!'

At this point I was joined by Rob, who wanted to know what the problem was and if I had abandoned them. I appealed to Rob to go back to Sandra and explained that I had a personal problem to sort out and I would join them shortly.

I'm sure Rob was thinking that I was a very strange man because of the way I was behaving but I did not want to tell him of my suspicions that we had been seated in a corner of the restaurant because of his wife's facial appearance or because of my disability!

As Rob returned to the restaurant, the deputy manager appeared and I was able to explain my suspicions. She assured me that my suspicions were all wrong and that there would have been a double-booking.

'I need evidence of that. So come with me now and show me on the booking plan that there has been a double booking,' I challenged.

'I'm far too busy. We have a maître d' to sort this kind of thing out.'

'I am not being put off. The Disability Discrimination Act prohibits what I suspect is happening to us. Could I give you the name of my solicitor, who will be contacting you?'

'Mr Counsell – there's no need for that. I'm sure we can find you another table in the restaurant. Just give me a moment to make a quick phone call.'

She walked away from me, presumably to her office, and returned a short time later to inform me that if I returned to the restaurant, Jenkins would find us another table. I assumed Jenkins was the maitre d' and I returned to Sandra and Rob.

We were reseated in the middle of the restaurant, but not in the centre, and we could enjoy our surroundings and the atmosphere much more than from our original corner.

The situation had to be explained to Rob and Sandra; they were oblivious to the fact that they had been discriminated against. Rob found it hard to believe and wanted to 'lay one on' the maître d' but quickly calmed down when Sandra assured him that I had dealt with the situation good and proper!

Actually, we did enjoy a wonderful meal and in my opinion the evening was a success, inasmuch as Sandra and I continued in cementing the relationship we had formed earlier when we met on the course and Rob and I got on well too. Rob wanted to talk about personal issues imposed on him by his wife's condition and he made comments about Sandra's personal development course. Eventually I steered the conversation away from disability and we shared a few laughs. Ironically no one sat at the table in the corner or any of the adjacent tables. Had I not challenged, we would have been isolated from the other diners and would have appeared very odd!

The icing on the cake was when we asked for the bill and we were told there was nothing to pay. The meal was on the house to compensate for any misunderstanding at the beginning of our evening.

This happened about fifteen years ago and Rob and Sandra still keep in touch with me. We meet up once or twice a year and reminisce and laugh about the experience at the restaurant when I first met Rob.

Sandra's condition did improve and she gradually returned to her former non-disabled self. Rob and Sandra now foster two children with disabilities, long-term, and I enjoy my role as surrogate uncle to those children.

I did hear, too, from the deputy manager of the hotel and through her contact, I was commissioned to design and deliver various training courses for the chain of hotels. My association with the deputy manager swelled the coffers of my company. The moral behind all this is that one never knows how a new acquaintance will impact on one's life!

***

I had strange things happening at home! Kathleen and I had always enjoyed a very close relationship in our marriage and I wasn't aware that we had any secrets. We shared everything. But suddenly Kathleen was receiving phone calls from a man who worked for a government department and who was supposed to be my friend. Sometimes he would call twice in one day and always, Kathleen would take his calls in private. She would say, 'Hang on a minute. Let me take this call in another room!' if I appeared while she was on the phone I would be asked to leave the room – she needed to 'take this call in private'.

It was frustrating for me and – but for the devilment in Kathleen's eyes and the sheer enjoyment which registered on her face as she assured me, 'Don't worry, everything will be explained eventually!' – I think there could have been a massive argument between us.

This behaviour went on for weeks and weeks and then I received a letter from the Leonard Cheshire Foundation informing me that I had been awarded an Enabled Award in the lifetime achievement category. I was dumbfounded – absolutely speechless.

This is what all the secret phone calls had been about. Kathleen had been helping my friend prepare the nomination for this award.

I felt incredibly honoured whilst at the same time embarrassed but I was also concerned. Before I could accept this award, I needed to know more about the award. If it had been awarded to me by non-disabled people, I didn't want it. I felt I was being patronised. I rang the Leonard Cheshire Foundation, spoke to the appropriate person and gave them a really hard time on the phone. Actually, I handled the situation wrongly out of embarrassment, I think, and I had to apologise later. It turned out that I had been nominated for the award by disabled people; not one non-disabled person had been involved in my nomination. I was embarrassed and I did not want to be patronised too!

***

In conclusion, I feel I am the richest man in the UK. I love my wife more than ever and we are really happy together. Kathleen and I enjoy relative good health and are able to enjoy life. We have a successful marriage and we are blissfully happy together. I am really proud of my children. They are successful, honest citizens who contribute to the community. I have a beautiful and talented daughter-in-law, who brings joy into my life, whilst my son-in-law is a treasure. I absolutely adore my five grandchildren; each is precious to me. I have friends who support me and make me feel of worth. My immediate neighbours are wonderful people and I enjoy my association with them. Throughout my life, I have contributed to society, I am proud to have worked all my life and I am and always have been independent. I have exceeded the expectations of my childhood. These are my riches. I reckon if one cannot get on with people then one is truly disabled!

So what next? Maybe it's time I retired and enjoyed a leisurely life. But I will continue to develop and grow – maybe into a grumpy old man, but I will continue to 'show them'.